Shifting Sands

Book Ten of the
Coming Back to Cornwall series

Katharine E. Smith

HEDDON PUBLISHING

First edition published in 2023 by Heddon Publishing.

ISBN Paperback 978-1-913166-79-3
ISBN Ebook 978-1-913166-78-6

Cover by Catherine Clarke Design
www.catherineclarkedesign.co.uk

www.heddonpublishing.com
www.facebook.com/heddonpublishing
@PublishHeddon

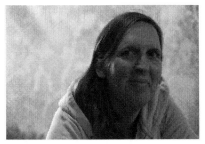

Katharine E. Smith is the author of sixteen novels, including the bestselling Coming Back to Cornwall series. Shifting Sands is the final book of this lovely series, which will be missed by readers and author alike.

A Philosophy graduate, Katharine initially worked in the IT and charity sectors. She turned to freelance editing in 2009, which led to her setting up Heddon Publishing, working with independent authors across the globe.

Katharine lives in Shropshire, UK, with her husband, their two children, and two excitable dogs.

You can find details of her books on her website:

www.katharineesmith.com

Information about her work with other authors can be found here:

www.heddonpublishing.com

and

www.heddonbooks.com

For my readers.

You have helped to make a dream come true!

Shifting Sands

"If one more person tells me that at least Mum and Dad are together again now, I will not be held accountable for my actions," Luke whispers into my ear. He has just shaken hands with an older man, and accepted a hug from the man's wife. Luke is smiling though, despite this, his face is drawn and sad.

"I can imagine," I say, putting my arm through his and squeezing gently. "Although I'm sure they mean well."

"Oh yeah, of course, I know. And I hope they're right, I really do, but… Heaven…? I don't know about all that… in fact, I think we just—"

"Daddy!" Before Luke has a chance to launch into his take on what happens to us when we die, Zinnia zooms into the room, and straight into Luke's arms.

"Hello beautiful," he smiles naturally this time, with genuine joy on his face.

"I went to the toilet!"

"Well, maybe you could say it a bit louder so the folk down the coast can hear," he grins.

Julie, following on, slips her arm around Luke's waist. "How are you doing?"

"Yeah, ok, I think. Just getting through it."

It's been a shock to us all. Whereas May, Luke's mum, had suffered a gradual decline in health, thanks to cancer, his dad's death had taken us all by surprise. Jim had recently begun working as a street pastor in Penzance, hoping to help people in need – whether a lone girl who had got separated from her friends on a night out, or talking things through with a sad, lonely drunk. Luke had been worried about his dad getting beaten up, or worse, but had not anticipated him being floored by a sudden heart attack during a leisurely stroll on a quiet, uneventful night.

Marie, Luke's sister, walks past us, looking determined and slightly hassled. Luke puts his hand out to her. "Stop, sis. Just stop for a minute."

Since arriving at their parents' house for the wake, Marie has been whizzing around, taking wraps off the platters of food, offering people drinks, clearing away plates and glasses... anything to keep busy, and avoid thinking about the reason for this gathering.

She looks at her brother and, almost immediately, tears spill from her eyes. I let go of Luke's arm and he draws her into a hug.

Julie steps in and takes the tray that Marie is awkwardly still clutching. "I'll take this," she says firmly. "Alice, can you take Zinnia to find Ben, do you think?"

"Of course. Come on, Zinnie. Let's go and find Ben and Holly, shall we? I think I know exactly where they'll be."

Zinnia slips her hand into mine and we head out through the conservatory, into the garden. I am reminded, not for the first time today, of May's funeral, when we were all so young. There was no Zinnia then – no Ben, no Holly. No me and Sam, either, or not quite. That was a beautiful summer's day, though, whereas now it's the tail end of winter, and the weather is neither here nor there. The day feels subdued, perhaps fittingly for this event, although I had so hoped that the sun would bless us with some brightness. I'm desperate for spring to break through and lighten up the world.

Beyond the house, and the trees, and down through the narrow streets of town, I know that the sea lies in wait, restlessly washing in and out, ready for its orders. At the top of one of the tall, dark conifers, a crow caws gloatingly down to me, while a gull struts its stuff on the rooftop, stopping to raise its head and shriek into the pale grey sky, announcing to all that Jim is gone.

I walk with his granddaughter to the end of the garden, and the little building which Luke and Marie had used as their teenage hangout, and where Sophie saw fit to hide one cold winter's night, in the throes of emotional upheaval – partly thanks to me. That was the night she had discovered Sam was not her 'real' dad. Life has moved on so far and so fast, I sometimes forget any of that happened.

I smile as I look through the window and catch sight of my little boy trying to show his little sister how to hold a pool cue. He has no chance. She just wants to wave it around, and I'm glad I arrive in time to stop her poking Ben's eye out.

"Shall I have that, Holly?" I ask, stepping through the door. She looks at me, annoyed, but hands it over. I smile. "Thank you. Zinnie and I were looking for you two. I had a feeling you'd be in here. Shall we get the Lego out?" I pull a huge box down from a low shelf. "I think it's a few years before you're big enough to play pool."

"Yes!" Ben shouts. "I love Lego!"

"I love Lego!" Holly copies.

"You're too young for Lego," he tells her. "You have Duplo."

I see Holly's bottom lip pout out, and I sit on the settee, drawing her towards me. Despite her frustration, she accepts my cuddle, and snuggles into me. "Tired?" I ask her.

"No," she says, pulling her thumb into her mouth and nestling her head against my shoulder.

"I didn't think so." I press a gentle kiss against her soft hair.

With a bit of effort, Ben and Zinnia tip the box of Lego onto the floor, and get stuck in. Ben attempts to manage proceedings, but Zinnia is having none of it.

"You get all the blue pieces," he says, "let's make a dragon."

"I don't want to make a dragon. I'm doing a shop."

I smile and sink back against the soft cushions, glad for a chance to just let things wash over me for a while.

The peace lasts for about ten minutes, until Zinnia looks out of the window. "Daddy's in the garden, and he's crying."

Her little face looks so sad. I go across and put my arm around her. I know she'll be finding all of this so hard, as much as the adults, even if she is able to turn on her play mode more easily.

I peer through the window, and see she's right. Sam is there, with his hand on Luke's shoulder, talking earnestly to him. I'm surprised to see Luke shake Sam's hand away. He picks up a wine bottle and refills his glass.

Sam says something, but Luke gives him a really harsh look, and Sam steps back, his hands up. I see Julie come out, and Luke turns his head away from her. She and Sam exchange a look. Now what do I do? I want to know what's going on, but I can't leave the kids here alone, and I know that if I set foot outside the door, Zinnia at least will want to come with me. I give her a little squeeze. "It's a sad time,

Zinnia. I'm sorry. It's very hard for all of you, and especially for your dad. But he wants to know that you're happy and having a nice time, so why don't you carry on with your building? What are you making again?"

"A shop."

"Oh yes, I can see that now. You carry on with that and maybe in a bit we can show Daddy." I glance out of the window again to see that Luke is now sitting alone, refilling his glass from that bottle of wine. "Or maybe we can show Mummy," I suggest.

Zinnia is already intent on her task, and she just nods. I sit back against the cushions again, but angled so I can keep an eye on the scene in the garden. Luke remains alone for a few minutes until Marie appears, and sits next to him. He is stiff and straight-backed for a moment, but she leans against him, and I see that he relents a little, then he puts down his wine glass and puts his arm around his sister. It's good to see, although it cuts an incredibly sad scene. I wonder what happened before. I will ask Julie when I get a chance but right now I am needed here, in this world of dragons and shops, and carefree make-believe.

1

I don't know if it's because I'm getting a bit older now, or whether it's an after-effect of covid, but it just feels like these days I know so many more people with health problems, with parents with health problems, or who have suffered the loss of a parent; both, in poor Luke's case. Looking back to the time that May died, it seemed like such freakish bad luck to lose a parent at such a young age, and of course it was. But these days, it's starting to feel almost like the norm. Now my generation have moved up a notch, and we're starting to feel the 'sandwich' effect. Looking after kids. Looking after parents. I have not escaped this myself, with Dad having never properly got over covid. He's not been himself, for some time.

"It's the way it goes though, isn't it?" Sam, ever-pragmatic, says when I voice these thoughts to him. We're sitting in our lounge, both kids asleep upstairs, and I've just returned from visiting my parents at the Sail Loft. "And these days, because modern medicine and science are keeping people alive for longer, it means that the middle-aged – don't pull that face, you've got to accept it, Alice, that's what we are – have to bear the burden of that. It's a double-edged sword."

Urgh! *Middle-aged.* Not me. I can't be. That is for my mum and dad. Except now, when I look at them, I know they are past that stage in their own lives. I can't quite bring myself to think of them as elderly, though, and I know they certainly don't consider themselves to be so, despite Dad's ongoing health struggles.

I'll be honest, I find it quite hard going to see them at the moment. Dad is not quite the man he used to be. He's so tired, and finds it hard to walk up the stairs – of which there are quite a few in the Sail Loft. He's had a load of tests, but they have been inconclusive, and the doctor has told him they think he's got long covid. Apparently that nasty, insidious, virus has caused some scarring on his lungs, and it's hard to see how he's really going to recover much further than he has already. Thank god Bea is managing the hotel for them – as I used to do for her.

Mum had pulled me aside, though, while Dad was making us some tea in the kitchen, having insisted on being the one to do so. "I'm worried about him, Alice."

That in itself hit me. There was a time that Mum would have protected me from any worries and concerns. Now she needs to share them with me. This is lovely in a way, and I'm so glad that she knows she can talk to me, but it's pushing me towards this new edge of reality, in which I have a great deal more responsibility. I mean, I'm a parent, and it doesn't really get much more responsible than that, but still, I often feel like I'm just making that up as I go along. I'm slowly beginning to realise that my own parents will have felt the same – and their parents before that. They weren't born parents, any more than I was.

"Does he actually rest when he needs to?" I asked Mum.

"Well, yes, he does – which is almost more worrying than

anything!" She offered a small laugh, but it nearly broke my heart. The creases on her face belied any humour in her remark.

"Yeah, that's not like Dad, is it?"

"But we've got this place to think about–" she gestured around the dark, wood-panelled hallway of the hotel – "and it's not easy, even with Bea. Well, you know how much work goes into keeping this afloat, and keeping it full, and keeping people happy. It's getting all the more expensive, too. I think that's worrying Phil as much as anything."

"It is all becoming a nightmare, isn't it?" I mused. "We've got the same problem at Amethi, too, but we've got to honour the prices for the people who've booked in advance. It's going to be a tight year." I generally try not to think too much about this, but I realise burying my head in the sand isn't going to help. Sometimes I am not even sure we can carry on, but I can't imagine a life without Amethi. I'm so grateful I have Julie to share these worries with.

"At least the weather should get better soon. No more need for heating."

"For a few months at least."

At that moment, Dad came out of the kitchen, pushing the swing door open with his back, making the crockery and cutlery shake a little on the tray.

"Here, Dad, let me take that." I easily swept the tray away from his hands and saw the look of annoyance cross his face – a bit like Holly's when I took the pool cue from her. I didn't want to patronise him, but he was clearly struggling.

I led the way into the little lounge, from where we could see the daylight was already vanishing, as though the sea

8

was greedily sucking it away, leaving a blank, empty sky for the night to do with as it pleased.

We sat and drank the tea quietly, each lost in contemplation. It was clear that Dad knew we'd been talking about him, which was painful. Then he and Mum both spoke at once.

"We can't keep on like this," were Dad's words, while Mum said, "We need to make a change, Phil."

"Well at least you're both thinking along the same lines," I said, mock-cheerfully. "But what do you mean, Dad?"

"I mean, we can't keep the Sail Loft," he said, matter-of-factly. "We can't afford it, financially, or for the sake of our health. It's not just me. You know your mum's had heart problems."

"Are you ill again, Mum?" I looked quickly at her, feeling an anxious clenching inside my own chest.

"No, no, I'm not, love. But your dad's right. All this stress can't be doing me any favours. I sometimes think we must have been mad, taking this on at our age."

"But… when you came here, things were different. There was no covid for a start," I protested.

"True, true. But I feel like I've aged fifteen years in the handful we've been at the Sail Loft. And that's not to say I don't love it. I really do, and I know you love it, too. But it's a young person's game. Bea already knew that; she stepped back when she was much younger than us."

"She had other things going on as well, though." Poor Bea, she'd met the love of her life – the tall, handsome Bob – and she'd left everything for him, and gone to live in the States, but he too had fallen victim to that bloody pandemic.

"She did," Mum agreed. "And I never, ever would wish on her what happened in her life, but I'm still so grateful she's here now. I think – I honestly believe – that we'd have gone under without her."

I relay all of this to Sam, who listens intently, and while he is listening, reaches out a hand to stroke the loose hair at the back of my neck. Sometimes, just sometimes – if I allow myself the chance to acknowledge it – I still get tingles from his gorgeous hands on my skin. It's good to know it's still there somewhere, amidst all the chaos and stress of being a parent and running a demanding business, and trying to help Mum and Dad, and keeping Karen and Ron involved in our lives... you get the picture. Life is good, but life is exhausting. Romance is not exactly a priority.

"That would be a real shame if they leave the Sail Loft – but I guess they can't run it forever. I think maybe your mum's right. It is a younger person's game," he says.

"But I don't want to think of them as old," I mock-wail.

"But... they sort of are." His kind eyes are looking at me with a slightly beseeching expression, asking me to accept it. While I am in partial denial about my parents getting older, he is very much accepting of the fact that his mum is progressing through life as she's meant to. Sometimes I think it's because he doesn't have the same kind of relationship with her that I do with my mum and dad; that maybe he doesn't care as much, but I know I'm wrong to think that way. It doesn't mean they love each other any less.

"I suppose I also don't like to think of the Sail Loft going to somebody else," I admit. "It's a huge part of me, and life here. My first job," I say wistfully.

"You did make a cute waitress," Sam says.

"Well thank you, I think. Though that sounds a little bit sexist to me..."

"Not sexist. Just honest."

"Hmm."

He leans forward and kisses me, and as I always do when we find a moment like this, I instantly recall the familiar, soft warmth of his mouth. I feel the tension melt just a little. Then, as he edges closer to me, and chances a hand on my waist, and then under my shirt, it melts a little bit more. I let my husband kiss me and pull me towards him and the stresses and strains of the day, and the day before, and the weeks and months before that, ebb blessedly away, just for a little while.

2

I'm finding it hard to concentrate today, my eyes being constantly drawn to the scene outside, where the sky is pelting rain unrelentingly down onto Amethi, and the rest of Cornwall – onto the whole of the UK, for all I know. It feels like it has rained forever, and my dreams of a soft, gentle spring easing us into summer are a thing of the past. Rain drips from the gutter above the window, and pools into the dips in the gravel of the paths and the car park. The ground is absolutely sodden, and our poor holiday-makers are at a loss as to what to do for the best. I have always been a great believer that the weather changes more frequently and more quickly by the sea, and I still think this is true, but it is very difficult to predict, and right now it doesn't feel like it will ever change again.

But I have to forget the weather. I need to keep my mind on work. There is so much to do this year – more than ever, and I've created a lot of the extra workload myself, but I really hope it is all going to be worth it.

Sighing, I take myself down the steep steps, in search of coffee. Lying by the door with her head on her paws, Meg looks as fed up as I feel. She gives a lacklustre wag of her tail at my approach. I crouch and stroke her and then I stand up, emitting that all-too familiar groan as my knees straighten and I roll my shoulders back.

"I know I'm old," I say to Meg. "Do you want to go out?"

Her ears prick up. She stands too, so that I can open the door, and we look at each other before we both step back at the miserable sight that greets us. It's not just the sight, but the sound as well. The constant battering of gravel and windows, and the wind pummelling its way through the trees.

"It's the apocalypse," I say to Meg, but she regards me wisely, as if to tell me to stop being so dramatic, and she simply lies back down, curling in on herself so that she's dry and warm as toast. I wish I could do the same.

In the kitchen, I put the kettle on and pluck a cafetière from the shelf. I put the kettle on to boil − not to boil, I remind myself, ever mindful of Julie's instructions as to how to make the perfect coffee: "Heat the water to just below boiling point − say ninety degrees. Add a scoop of coffee per cup, and pour the water in gently, from a low height, in a circular motion. Get a spoon − plastic, not metal − and stir it around gently until the crema is swirling slowly around on the surface. Then let it brew for a few minutes before you plunge."

Yeah, yeah, Julie. Still, I do as she says. I heat some oat milk in the microwave (not the pan, just to show that I don't do everything Julie tells me) and pour it into one of the thick, cream-coloured jugs. I plunge the coffee and I put the cafetière, jug, and a couple of small packs of biscuits on a tray, then take it all upstairs and close the office door behind me. Now I am set with provisions and have no excuses not to crack on with my work. Besides, there is much I have to do before Julie arrives.

I'm not used to keeping secrets from my best friend, but it's for a good cause. This is a year of anniversaries, you see. Not just anniversaries, which of course happen every year, but tenth anniversaries. It's ten years since we took on Amethi. And it's ten years since Julie and Luke got married – David and Martin, too. I was vaguely aware of this, of course, but my mind was on Amethi, as Julie and I have been planning a celebration of our decade here since last summer.

Then Bea suggested we might need a further celebration, for David and Martin, and that we might try and make it a surprise. Bea, whose own tenth wedding anniversary occurred in the autumn, but who had to find her way through it without her husband. Somehow, she still has the generosity of spirit to want to celebrate her brother's happiness.

This got me thinking, about Julie and Luke, and the tough times they've had over their years together, with both of Luke's parents having died, and the hard time they had trying to conceive. Julie would say that was all meant to be, and I know without a doubt that Zinnia is Julie's and Luke's daughter, the biology of it just a small and largely irrelevant detail. Nevertheless, after all the difficult times, I feel that we need to celebrate everything we possibly can and so, as well as well as helping Bea plan David and Martin's surprise party, which thankfully is not until New Year's Eve, I've decided that I will arrange a celebration for Julie and Luke, too. All of which is not necessarily straightforward, as Julie and I are working together on the Amethi celebration in the summer – and also David and Martin's – and there is inevitably some crossover with suppliers. I'm worried that one of them will manage to give the game away. At least Lydia has agreed to host the Julie and Luke party at the Bay Hotel, as I'd find it impossible to hide an Amethi event from Julie. No matter what cunning way I devised to disguise it, she'd know something was up. I don't think I'm the best at keeping secrets, or at least not without arousing suspicion. When we are both in the office, I regularly snatch the phone up before Julie has a chance to answer, and I know she thinks I've been being weird.

I have just under two hours before Julie is due to arrive, and there is much to do. I'm worried, as well, that she and Luke might not even want this. They might very well just want to do their own thing. They could book themselves a holiday, although they can't do that without me knowing, as Julie and I have to sort out any extraordinary leave between us. Plus, Zinnia is at school now, and Julie has surprised me by how much of a rule-follower she is when it comes to her daughter's education (she certainly was not like that when she and I were at school), so I doubt they would plan anything during term-time. I therefore have opted for the weekend before the autumn half-term break when, if the last few years have been anything to go by, there is a good chance of some warmth in the day, and maybe even some sunshine, although this is not guaranteed by any means.

With our Amethi celebration party in early September, and David and Martin's surprise party planned for New Year's Eve, there is just a couple of months between each, and although it is only spring, I know time will fly by, especially with a nearly fully-booked Amethi all the way through the year.

I pour a large mug of coffee and take a sip, marvelling at the immediate warmth that spreads through me. Although the office is heated, I feel chilly, and my hands are apt to make careless errors when they're cold. They can't always keep up with the thoughts in my head.

I open the spreadsheet I have saved in my 'Poetry' folder, knowing that Julie is very, very unlikely to have her interest piqued by that name. I have a list of guests to invite, and all their contact details. A separate sheet on the file has all the names of bands I am contacting for a quote. The next one has food suppliers – which is possibly the most important thing where Julie is concerned. Usually, whenever we have a celebration, this side of things is covered by her of course, and guests never fail to be impressed by her skill and attention to detail. I want the same for her, and I'm floundering a bit. I can't even ask Luke for ideas, because this is a secret from him, too.

"Are you sure you haven't bitten off more than you can chew, Alice?" Sam has asked me more than once, and I've almost bitten his head off in reply.

"It will be worth it," I say through gritted teeth, trying to convince myself as much as him.

"If you say so." And, Sam being Sam, he's game to help out if I need him to. I've tasked him with making sure Luke and Julie are free the weekend of the party, so that at least is one thing I don't have to worry about. Although, Julie being Julie, she keeps asking what we're planning. Maybe I need to plant a few false clues around the place. As if I've got time for that!

Today, I need to go through the emails I've got in the

account I have set up specifically for this party, and see if anyone new has responded to the invites. Julie's mum Cherry did, immediately, as did my parents – even though I'd already mentioned it to all of them and I knew they were coming. Karen has responded verbally for her and Ron, so with me, Sam, Ben, Holly and Zinnia as well, that makes at least nine of us. Out of the hundred I have invited.

"A hundred!" Sam nearly spat out his cornflakes. "We don't know that many people!"

"Well, actually… between Luke and Julie, it's not even everyone I could think of." There are a handful of schoolfriends whom neither Julie nor I have seen in years but who I know it will be lovely to see again. Of course, I couldn't invite them without their partners and kids. There is Julie's cousin Lucy and her partner, India. Luke's sister Marie, of course, and her family. Also Lee, Julie's brother – and his on-again-off-again girlfriend Nicole, if they are on-again at the time. Bea and David and Martin, plus Tyler and Esme, and then there's Lizzie – with her sort-of boyfriend Med, if he's around. Cindy, who cleans at Amethi, and her husband Rod. Some of our suppliers, who have come to be friends over the years. Sophie, of course, and by extension Kate, Isaac and Jacob, although they are likely to be too busy running their own place in Devon to be able to come down. Paul Waters, and Shona – who I must speak to again about the PR for our Amethi party. I make a note to call her.

I've invited some of Luke and Sam's schoolfriends as well, including Christian from the Cross-Section – who may also be providing the food, but I really want him to come as a guest in his own right. He and Luke and Sam have been friends for years.

I am so worried that somebody will let something slip about this, and Sam has suggested I just tell Julie and Luke that I'm planning a party, but not give them any details.

"You're missing the point!" I said. "Anyway, remember when you sprang the surprise party for me?"

"Surprise *wedding*," he reminded me.

"Yes, surprise wedding!" I had stopped for a moment to consider and appreciate everything Sam had done, after we'd had to cancel our original wedding plans. "My god, that was amazing! It meant so much, that you'd done it all without me knowing. I want to do the same for Julie and Luke. It's a lovely feeling."

"Just as long as you don't do anything like this for me," he said. "I do not like surprises. And no, I am not saying that but secretly hoping you'll plan one for me. I really, truly, do not want a surprise party. Ever."

"Understood."

Checking my inbox, I see that David has replied, and so has Shona. I add them to the list headed 'Yes', along with Martin, Tyler and Esme for David, and Paul for Shona.

I also have an email from Skaburst, a favourite band of Luke's and Julie's, who say they will come down from Telford for it.

"Yes!" I shout, surprising myself.

"Won the lottery?" I hear Julie say as the door opens. Shit. I didn't hear her come in. I clumsily fumble to close down the spreadsheet but, having not saved my changes, a little box pops up on screen, asking me if I want to. Hopefully, I have managed to confirm that yes I do want to, before Julie has seen anything. I feel a flush rising up my neck towards my face.

Julie gives me a weird look. "Everything alright?"

"Oh, yeah, I was just… I just got those numbers to add up, you know, the income and outgoings I was messing about with."

"Er… no, but sounds fascinating."

I am not sure she believes me, but never mind.

"What are you doing here so early, anyway?"

"Ah well, just… lots to do, you know."

I realise Julie looks a little bit uncomfortable herself. "Is everything OK?"

"Yeah… well… no… Well, sort of."

"Luke?"

"Yeah." She sits down on her desk chair with a bit of a bump. And she looks thoroughly glum. "He's just in such a bad way. Which is totally understandable; of course it is. But – and I will be honest with you, Alice, because it's you – he's bloody hard work. I know, I know, that's a horrible thing to say. His dad's just died. I'm a terrible person."

"You're not, Julie. You're really not!" I put my hand on hers. "It's just hard. Life is hard sometimes. I know you're supporting him, and looking after Zinnia, and working your arse off here... And I also know that Luke has to get through this part of his life somehow, but that doesn't necessarily work very well with what you're trying to do."

When I did get a chance to ask Julie what had happened back at Jim's house after the funeral, she told me that she'd suggested Luke stop drinking. It had not gone down well. "I just wanted him to wake up the next day with a clear head, not a raging hangover. And also, he was getting dangerously close to telling his uncle Graham what he really thinks of him. But he accused me of judging him, and said I had no idea what he is going through. Which is partly true, of course, but I wasn't judging... just trying to support him, and make sure he didn't do anything he'd regret later."

Sam had apparently come to Julie's aid and tried to make Luke see sense but of course this also did not go down well. Hence the scene I had witnessed in the garden.

"If anything, it probably made him drink even more," Julie acknowledged. "You know how he hates being told what to do."

"Well, yes," I said, "but I thought Luke had his head screwed on better than that. Still, I have no idea what it feels like to lose a parent, never mind two. I don't suppose it's very easy to keep a straight head when everything's so raw."

Now Luke has cancelled his work for a couple of weeks, and I already know from Sam that he's not been answering his phone, or responding to any messages. I know Luke, and that he is usually such an upbeat and warm person, but I also know it's not fair or realistic to expect him to always be that way. He was so close to his dad, he must be going through hell right now. He can't just put a brave face on it.

But I can see how hard this is for Julie. I've certainly seen Sam go into a slump more than once, when to outsiders, and at work, I expect he seemed his usual happy, friendly self. It is horrible feeling awful, but it is also not easy to live with somebody in that kind of state; even less so when you've got young children.

"Alice, I knew you'd get it. Thank you. And this is why I've come into work early. Not to work, but to drink coffee and talk to you!" Her eyes take in the cafetière. "Any of that left?"

"There is, but it's not very warm – shall I make you a fresh one? Let's go down to the kitchen, shall we? I could do with a break from the office."

"Spreadsheets will do that to you," Julie agrees, and I breathe an internal sigh of relief. It looks like I might just have got away with my little white lie.

3

It's just too wet to sit outside with the coffee, and I can't wait for the day that we can do that again. I know it's coming but it really doesn't feel like it. It has to be coming, doesn't it? It can't really rain forever. I imagine closing my eyes, the feeling of the sun on my face. Just thinking about it makes me smile.

Instead, we sit inside the Mowhay, at the end of the long dining table.

"Cheers." Julie raises her mug to mine.

"Cheers. Now, tell me about Luke."

"Nah, it's boring."

"Well, yeah, obviously it's boring," I am pleased to see her mouth curl into a small smile, "but you need to let it all out. Release some of the steam."

"Thanks, Alice. I think there's a lot of steam. And it's all so mixed up in here," she gestures to her own head. She's as beautiful as ever, my friend, but I can see the strain on her face. And the tiredness in her eyes. I stay quiet, and let her continue at her own pace. "Like, I absolutely one hundred per cent know that Luke is in a bad place. He's been through an awful time, and he's missing his dad, and feeling so incredibly awful. Which means I don't feel like I can say anything. I can't say that I know how he feels. Not really. I've still got Mum, and Dad has never really been part of my life anyway. I know Luke needs space, and time. But equally, we've got Zinnie, and she needs us, and she's missing Jim, too. I feel like she's missing Luke as well. I know I am."

"Poor Luke," I say. "Poor all of you."

"Urgh. I hate it. I miss Jim too, of course, but there's something so deep in losing your own parents, I think. If you're lucky to have parents who care, anyway. Maybe even if they're crap parents. Even then, when they're gone, suddenly you're alone in the world."

"But Luke isn't alone," I say, although I know what she means.

"He's the top generation as well now, isn't he? No more barriers between him and his own mortality."

"I hope he's not thinking like that."

"Maybe not consciously, but it's a natural thought process, I reckon."

"Would he see a counsellor, do you think?"

"I don't know. I've mentioned it, tentatively. I don't think he feels like it will help."

"Hmm." I can see that. Luke isn't necessarily the type to want to open up to a stranger. "I think Sam would be the same."

"But I am so poorly qualified to get him through this." Unusually, Julie's eyes fill with tears, which she wipes away with irritation.

"Oh, Julie. I don't know. You will get through it. People do. Which doesn't make it any easier while you're right in the middle of it, but I know you'll find a way through. And Luke, too. He probably needs a big blow-out in a way.

23

Should I ask Sam to organise something? Just the two of them? A day's walking, and a night's drinking? Actually, maybe not the drinking. Sorry."

"That sounds amazing. He might just go for it."

"And maybe you should think about counselling for yourself, if Luke isn't up for it. Or even if he is. It might help you work your way through this. You were close to Jim as well. Don't belittle your relationship with him because Luke's claim on him is larger."

"You know, I think I do feel like that. You're pretty smart sometimes, you know."

"Only sometimes, though."

"Yes, just occasionally."

I shuffle my chair across so I can put my arm around her shoulder, and so she can lean her head against me. We sit like that for a few minutes, not talking. I can hear Julie's breathing, and the rain and the wind outside. Meg's claws scratch the hard floor as she stands and turns around a couple of times before lying down again.

I close my eyes. Sometimes, in quiet moments like this, I think I can feel the spirit of this place. Perhaps that should be spirits, plural. Right now, I imagine them breathing quietly, tiptoeing around us as they go about their business, or perhaps just sitting and watching, contemplating the two of us. The caretakers of Amethi.

After a while, we straighten up, and finish our coffees. Julie and I are very much in tune with one another, as I suppose we should be after all this time.

"Thank you, Alice," Julie says. "I do actually feel a little bit better now."

"Good. Now, I hate to say this, because what's going on with you guys is so much more important, but shall we have a look at some work stuff?"

"Of course. I think it would do me good to get my head into something different."

"Great. Well, let's start with the bills, shall we?"

"If we have to." Julie mock-sighs.

"Then we can move on to our birthday celebrations. That seems like the right way round."

"Agreed. Come on then, let me have it."

I pull my phone from my pocket and log in to the Amethi utilities account.

"Shit!" Julie says.

"I know."

We have been hit hard, as has every small business, and every household, by the huge hike in gas and electricity prices. And because the weather has been so appalling, our guests have not only been staying in their holiday accommodation more than they might normally, but they've also been making good use of the heating and electricity, as is their right and as is totally understandable. But it's going to cut deep into our profits this year. It's another reason I am desperate for some better, brighter weather.

"We just have to take the hit with it, but we can't do that more than once. I think we seriously need to review our pricing."

"Which is difficult, when we've got so many return guests."

"Yes, but I think they'll understand. They kind of have to."

"I know. And we need to take food prices into account as

well. They've properly shot up. I just hope it doesn't put people off coming."

I'm scared, to be honest, about how or whether we will be able to carry on as we are doing. This has always been a bit of a luxury place, with the extra service Julie and I offer in terms of catering, and booking excursions, events, etc. There are of course people out there still well able to afford luxury, but they are fewer and further between. And now we're going to have to hike our prices up, they will be even harder to find. Still, Julie has enough on her mind, and I feel like I need to ease the pressure on her in terms of work – for the time being, at least. "I think we're all in the same boat. We can't be the only ones having to do this. And it's been a while since we've increased our pricing. People will know it's not just us being greedy."

"I just hope it's sustainable, Alice. I really do."

That worn expression has returned to my friend's face. Of course she's worrying in the same way that I am. I think of Mum and Dad with similar problems at the Sail Loft, plus Dad's health issues, and paying Bea's wages. Is any of this sustainable, really? Time will tell, I suppose.

Still, right now it is important to keep things as positive as possible. I want to take the strain from Julie for a while. "We'll run it past the accountants and see what they think, and take it from there. Don't worry, I'll get in touch with them, and maybe we can get them in next week to go through it all. Now, let's move on to something a bit more cheerful. Our tenth birthday!"

"I can't believe it's been ten years! Being here, or being married. God, it makes me feel old."

"I know exactly what you mean. But also… ten years! We have made this work for ten years! And we've barely had an argument. I think that in itself is something worth celebrating!"

"That is certainly true. And I know I haven't been pulling my weight enough in getting this party sorted, so tell me where we are, and what to do now. I need to take some of this off your hands."

"OK, let me go and get my laptop, and I'll show you what's what." We could go up to the office, but I'm enjoying sitting in the Mowhay, despite the dismal weather on full display through the bifold doors and windows. Also, this will give me the chance to make sure that the 'Poetry' folder on my computer is definitely closed.

I give Meg a little rub as I pass her, and she rumbles a little in appreciation, but barely bothers to open her eyes. She's greying on her cheeks now, and, while I don't know quite how old she is, it's clear that age is catching up with her. Something else I don't want to think about. Why can't dogs live as long as we do?

Upstairs, I wake up my laptop and open up the '10th Anniversary' folder. I have a similar spreadsheet in here to the one I've got for the surprise party, so if I open that up, if Julie had seen anything on my computer when she came upstairs, hopefully she'll assume it was this same spreadsheet. I am probably being far too careful; I know Julie wilfully banishes all thoughts of Excel from her mind if she can.

I close the laptop and walk carefully down the steep stairs. As I round the corner into the Mowhay, I see Julie is intently tapping out a message into her phone, so I stay still for a moment until it looks like she's finished.

"Here we go," I say, announcing my presence. She tucks her phone into her pocket, and I walk across, putting the laptop on the table and sitting down so that we can both see the screen. Even though I know I've opened the right spreadsheet, I still experience a moment of panic that it's the secret one. But all is well.

"So here are the entertainment options," I say.

"Skaburst can't do it?" she asks, disappointed.

"Sadly not," I say, hiding my smile and allowing myself a moment's satisfaction, that I've secured them for her and Luke's party instead. "However, we can have Half a Pint of Shanty. Should we?"

"Yes, go on then!" Julie grins. Our local shanty singers are always good fun and I think more fitting for our Amethi party anyway. Everyone will enjoy them, I am sure of it.

"Hello, hello!" I hear Meg get to her feet as the door opens and Lizzie comes in, to be greeted by a joyful dog. She surveys the scene before her: Julie, me, a laptop, and a sheaf of papers. "Am I interrupting something?"

"Well, just party-planning, actually."

"Oh yeah?" Lizzie is in on my plan for the surprise party, but I know she's not going to give anything away.

"Yes, I think we've got our band sorted."

"Brilliant! Who are you having?"

We tell her, and she smiles. She's friends with a couple of the shanty singers, from way back. "That's very fitting."

"I thought so!" I grin. "Now we need to decide on caterers, and drink suppliers. The trouble is, everyone's so expensive."

"Tell me about it."

28

I notice Lizzie is looking less relaxed than normal. "Is everything OK?" I ask.

"Yes… well, sort of. I mean, actually, quite exciting, but…"

"Spit it out!" says Julie.

"Med's asked me to join him." Lizzie is unable to suppress her smile as she says this. "In France. And to travel round Europe in his van."

"Oh wow!" I exclaim. "That's fantastic, Lizzie."

"It is, isn't it? But…"

"But you won't be in Cornwall," Julie fills in.

"No."

"So we won't have you with us anymore?" I ask, though it's a pretty pointless question.

"I'm so sorry, but no. If I could be in two places at once, I would. You know I love it here, and I love you guys, but…"

"Don't say another word, Lizzie! I mean, we love you too, of course we do, but this is brilliant. A proper adventure. And nice to spend more time with Med." All of this is true. And Lizzie deserves it. Despite all the amazing times she has worked with us, she does not work for Amethi directly. There was always going to be a chance that she wanted to move on and do something new.

"It will be nice to spend more time with him," she says, with that smile again. "And to travel. I've been getting restless, I knew there was something afoot."

"So don't give Amethi, or us, a second thought," says Julie. "Think of all the amazing places you're going to see. You can't pass up an opportunity like this."

"Oh thank you, guys. I was dreading telling you. And you

know I really do love it here, and working with you both, and the retreats, and…"

Her eyes are gleaming, and her happiness is self-evident. It's impossible not to be pleased for her.

I remember my first meeting with Lizzie, and how I'd worried she wouldn't fit in with what Julie and I were doing, but she has been perfect for us and for Amethi. The guests have all loved her, and she's opened my mind to so much more about life, and the world, than I could have imagined.

I can't help but think about the business side of things, though, because we have yoga retreats booked until the end of the year. I don't want to ask about this right now, because it feels like I'd be raining on her parade, but it's something we will have to discuss. I know it will be on Julie's mind, too. I suppose this was always going to be a problem eventually, working with somebody like Lizzie, who is not overly keen on being tied to things. It's a necessity for our business, to plan ahead and know what's coming up, but for Lizzie that is probably the polar opposite of how she likes to live her life. Still, she's paid well for the work she does here. But we've never had a contract as such – it didn't feel right somehow. And despite this potential problem looming, I stand by that.

"I know we've got retreats booked in this year," Lizzie says, as though reading my mind. "I've told Med this, too. I don't know what to do, to be honest. He will wait for me, till September, till after the equinox. But he wants to be on the move before winter. To be honest, so do I."

"Okay…" Julie says, as she thinks things through. "Okay. Well, that gives us some time, doesn't it? And are all the retreats booked, Alice?"

"Actually, the winter one isn't, fully – I think there's just three on that one so far."

"OK. So maybe we put a hold on advertising it, for the time being, and we try to find somebody who can fill Lizzie's shoes."

"Impossible!" I say, standing and hugging Lizzie. Her wild hair tickles my nose.

"Ha! They'll be out there somewhere. I've got a couple of ideas," Lizzie says, "but it's got to be someone who feels right for you."

Which sounds more straightforward than it is. But we will come to that. Just another thing to add to the Amethi to-do list. There is some time to find the right person before winter – if only there weren't another hundred-plus other things to do in the meantime.

"Honestly, Lizzie, that sounds really exciting," Julie says, standing to hug Lizzie as well. "You'll have to stay in touch, and let us know where you are – maybe we can meet up somewhere sometime. On our winter break!"

"That would be really fantastic," Lizzie grins, and despite the work concerns, I genuinely can't feel anything other than delighted for her.

My phone begins to buzz on the table. I pick it up and look at the screen. "Oh no."

"Who is it?"

"Nursery," I whisper, as I answer the call. "Hello?"

"Hi, Alice? This is Lisa. Sorry to bother you."

"That's OK, it's no bother at all."

"It's just Holly doesn't seem her normal self. We think maybe she's coming down with something."

"Oh no, really?" This is all I need, I think, and then kick myself for thinking of my daughter's wellbeing as an inconvenience. I don't mean it, of course. I just wish that I could have a clear day to get through some of this work. And make a plan. It feels like everything is up in the air, and like I am doing nothing as well as I would want to.

"Yes, she's a bit drowsy," Lisa explains, "and she says her legs are aching. Maybe it's something fluey? A few of the children have had sniffles lately."

"When don't they?" I laugh. "Alright, I'll come and get her."

I look apologetically to Julie, who smiles and shrugs. We both have to do this from time to time. I can always bring Holly here if she's not too bad.

"Sorry, both of you, I'm going to have to run. But I might be back."

"No worries," says Julie. "I think we're getting there anyway, with the party. Is there anything I need to know about this evening? Just in case you don't make it back. Menu changes, that kind of thing?"

"Nope, all is as requested." We've got a large group of friends at Amethi this week; young families, the parents were all friends with each other at school or at uni, I think. Making the most of term-time holidays while they can. I feel sorry for them that the weather's not great, but there's definitely nothing I can do about that.

"Do you want me to man the phones?" Lizzie offers.

"Actually, if you don't mind, Lizzie, that would be wonderful. I'll let you know if Holly's feeling really awful. Otherwise, I'll be back in half an hour or so."

"No problem. Why don't you leave Meg, too? Seems a shame to rouse her!"

We all look fondly at the sleeping dog, who seems to feel our attention on her and opens an eye, surveying us briefly before flopping onto her side and continuing her slumber.

"OK, if you're sure. Thank you!"

I shut my laptop and go up to the office to get my bag, then I pull on my coat and, hood up, I half-run across the soaking gravel to the car park, feeling the dampness seep through my well-worn boots and putting my coat into the back of the car before I get into the driver's seat, by which time by shoulders are already drenched.

Windscreen wipers going double-speed, I bump slowly along the driveway and exit through the line of trees, heading out into the rest of the world.

4

"Mummy!" Holly is in Lisa's arms, but she immediately holds hers out to me, and I take her, pulling her body close to mine. She wraps her little legs around me and I'm struck, as I often am these days, that it might not be too long before I'm unable to hold her like this. She's growing up. And soon she'll be at school, with Ben. There's no holding back time, so I just have to try and hold on to these moments, and remember these feelings. Besides, as I am discovering with Ben, it's exciting seeing children grow up and learn new things, gaining confidence and independence.

"Sorry to call you at work, Alice," Lisa says.

"It's absolutely fine. Looks like you've been having an eventful day!" Her nursery-logo sweatshirt is covered with flour.

"Ha! Yes. Every day. I do love it, though."

"Well, Holly loves you too, and we're all really grateful for how well you look after her." I hold Holly a little away from me so I can take a look at her. She too has a liberal coating of flour, but little tear-tracks have run through it on her cheeks. "Ahh, poor girl. You feeling poorly?"

Holly just nods her head, sorry for herself.

"Come on then, let's get you home, shall we?" Although I'd thought I might take her to Amethi, it doesn't feel fair, really. Not on Holly, and not on Julie or Lizzie, if Holly's got a bug. If I'm honest, the thought of taking my little girl home and snuggling on the sofa with her, maybe watching a bit of CBeebies, is very appealing. I carry her across to the car and decide to head through town to pick up some Calpol, but before we've even made it to the station car park, I can see her head is lolling forward with sleep.

I drive on down to the harbour, which in the summer months is teeming with tourists, milling along the promenade and spilling into the road, holding up the drivers – who already have a struggle on their hands to navigate their way around the town and find a parking spot. Today, though, there is barely a soul about, and those who have braved this further downpour are wrapped up in waterproofs, hoods pulled over their heads, shoulders hunched but striding determinedly along, attempting to avoid the puddles. The rain is creating a mist above the sea, which is all the way in at the moment, hiding the sand that people often walk across at low tide. It feels like an entirely different town to that of the high season and, although I really do wish it would stop raining sometime soon, I feel privileged to see it like this.

Around the harbour, I follow the little side streets which bring me to the Island car park. I pull into an empty space facing the sea, and turn the engine off. Holly is now snoring gently in the back, and I look at her pale face, and the slight, delicate blue veins of her eyelids. Not for the first time, I experience a pang of guilt that I palm her off to a nursery, for somebody else to look after her while I go to work. I know it's stupid, and that this is something so many parents do (and that so many feel the same way I do), but sometimes, when I'm contemplating how short childhood really is, I think that I'm wasting this time I could be spending with my children. And while Lisa and the others at Goslings are fantastic, it doesn't make it any easier.

Still, on the flipside, as many people tell me – very often Lizzie – for Ben and Holly to see their mum working hard and being successful is a positive.

"It's a very powerful thing," Lizzie has told me more than once. "Honestly, and look what it is you're doing, as well. Your ethos at Amethi is great. And you're always there for the kids when they need you – Sam is, too. You've got a balance, Alice. That's what it's all about."

I appreciate all of this, and I can imagine myself saying the same thing to somebody else, but when it's yourself you're critically examining, it's a bit different, isn't it?

Now, I sit back for a while and let Holly sleep. My gaze wanders outside, greedily taking in the details of the scene before me, all of which are softened and shaded by the constant drizzle. If I turn my head far enough, I can see at the top of the Island that beautiful little chapel, where my old workmate Stef got married. He has long since gone back to Sweden, taking his family with him. We made the usual promise to keep in touch and visit each other, but so far have not quite managed either very well. Family life and work take up nearly all of my energy, and I imagine it's the same for him. Still, I know it's a mistake to just assume we'll get round to it someday. The days go fast, and soon we're racking up the years.

Down from the car park is the little middle beach, as I

think of it, with its colourful wooden huts and lovely little café. I'd love to go in; sit in the window to drink in this view, but I need to keep Holly asleep, and I couldn't really drag her in there when she's poorly anyway, so the car will have to do. A coffee wouldn't go amiss, though.

In front of me, just visible through my windscreen, which is still being rapidly and repeatedly cleared by the windscreen wipers, is an outcrop of rocks, where a cormorant huddles disconsolately. The sea itself has taken on the colour of the sky; a deep, dark grey. It is unsettled, but not wild. Just, perhaps, waiting for spring to actually kick in − like the rest of us are. My mind drifts to what is below its murky surface; what secrets lie on the sands down there, and what creatures are moving sleekly and silkily through the depths. There have been local sightings of dolphins and even whales, more frequently than ever before. Days last summer when the sands were covered with poor stranded jellyfish. The waters are warming, though somebody might like to remind me of that when I go for an early morning swim. It's still not like the sea in Thailand, which I remember very fondly − and sometimes longingly − from my long-ago trip there with Sam. That kind of holiday is a thing of the past for us. Perhaps a thing of the future, too − although only a very distant future, I suspect.

In the back of the car, Holly stirs. I need to get her home. I message Sam:

Holly's poorly. I've picked her up and we're on our way home. Could you get some Calpol on your way back please? Xx

Then I message Mum:

Is there any chance you could get Ben after school please? He's doing a club so he won't need collecting till four. Holly's ill so I'm taking her home xx

Then I reverse out of the parking space, being extra careful to check for unexpected pedestrians, cars or bikes looming out of the rain, and drive up past the surf beach, rounding the cemetery, then we're back at our house within minutes. I check my phone for messages.

Sam: **Oh no, is she ok? Are you? Can you manage workwise? And no probs about the Calpol, let me know if we need anything else x**

Mum: **I'm so sorry, Alice, I'm at the doctors with your dad this afternoon. Can you ask Karen? Hope H is ok xxx**

I will ask Karen, and not mention to her that I'd asked my mum first. It makes me feel a bit guilty, thinking like this, but I know Karen sometimes feels a bit pushed out. I don't want her to, and I need to get better at thinking of her.

First, though, I will get Holly into the house. She murmurs as I pick her up, and she feels a bit clammy to the touch. I pull my coat off and wrap it around her for the short dash through the rain to the front door, which thankfully has a small porch around it as respite from the weather.

I have to dig deep in my pocket for the key, while still supporting Holly. I've become quite adept at this over the years, though, and we are soon in.

Damn, I've left Meg at Amethi. I'd better ask Sam to collect her as well on his way back.

There are so many things to think about, I can feel my heart start to beat more rapidly sometimes as I contemplate all that I have to do, and remember, and achieve. All the responsibilities I have. I just hope Karen can help with Ben. I unwrap the coat from around Holly and I take her through to the lounge, where I place her on the settee, and she immediately grabs her soft elephant blanket which she'd left there this morning.

"Are you alright, Holly? Do you need anything?"

"Drink please, Mummy," she says, already reaching for the TV remote, which she expertly uses with one hand, the other busily clutching her blanket.

"OK. No problem."

As I go into the kitchen, I hear the sound of some kids' cartoon that Ben likes. Already, he's moving on and away from CBeebies, and Holly, who would like to do everything he does, is following.

I put the kettle on to boil, and make Holly a cup of squash. She gulps it down quickly and asks for another.

"You are thirsty!" I say. "It won't do you any harm to get some fluids into you, though."

I'm relieved to see that she seems to have a little more colour in her cheeks. Sometimes, we just need to be at home. The kettle clicks off as I go back into the kitchen, so I fish a herbal tea bag from the jar and put it in a mug, pouring the hot water over it and breathing in the fragrant steam. Then I refill Holly's cup and take it back to her. She drinks greedily. Then, "Need a wee," she says.

"I'm not surprised! Off you go, then."

"Carry me, Mummy!"

"You don't need carrying, do you? You're a big girl now, you can go yourself."

Her mouth turns down and I see tears threatening. "My legs hurt."

"Do they, lovely?" Oh no, I'm thinking, it might be covid. That particular little bugger has not yet properly left us, if indeed it ever will, and if I'm honest I am always half expecting it to make some kind of dramatic return.

"Alright." I give in, as I'm pretty sure Holly knew I would. I scoop her up, blanket and all, and take her through to the toilet, where I hold the blanket for her while she sorts herself out and settles on the seat. She is normally extremely chatty while she's on the toilet but today she just sighs. She does look tired. Poor little thing. I'm glad I've brought her home, rather than dragging her up to Amethi.

She manages the long, arduous walk back to the settee without being carried, then climbs onto the seat, pulls the blanket back over herself, and curls up. I retrieve my mug from the kitchen, then realise I've left my laptop in the car. Never mind. It can wait a while. I must message Karen, though.

When I sit down next to Holly, she changes position so that she's resting against me. It feels very nice, and cosy, just the two of us.

I bring out my phone and send Karen a message:

Hi Karen, are you busy this afternoon? I was just wondering if you were able to collect Ben from school at four please? Holly's home ill and I want to avoid dragging her out if I can. xx

A message pings back nearly straightaway:

Sorry, Alice. Elaine's just asked me to the cinema. They're doing an afternoon screening of Casablanca, and we're having tea afterwards too. If you'd asked me half an hour ago I'd have said yes. Hope Holly's OK. Big kiss to her and Ben xx

Well that serves me right, doesn't it? I could ask Luke, as he'll be collecting Zinnia, but she might not be in an after-school club and be going home at the normal time. Besides, after what Julie's told me, I think perhaps Luke doesn't need anyone asking him for favours at the moment.

We will just have to go in the car and get Ben. It's not the end of the world. There is still an hour or so before we need to leave so I can settle in for a bit and enjoy this time with Holly. Maybe she'll be feeling a bit better after a rest.

5

"Hi Alice, how's Holly?" I hear Mum's cheerful voice ask. And yet, there is something not quite right. I know Mum. That cheeriness conceals a slight shake. *Dad!* I think, kicking myself. I hadn't forgotten they had that appointment this afternoon – well, I had, as illustrated when I asked Mum if she could pick Ben up from school – but it's not been at the forefront of my mind. It's in there, somewhere, muddled up with all the thousand and one other things I've got to remember, or sort through, or problem-solve.

"She's OK thanks, Mum. I think she's just got a bug." She had been alright, when we went to get Ben. She chatted away to me on our way to the school, and she gave Ben a huge hug when he came out. I was happy to see he looked pleased and a bit proud of this, rather than embarrassed. Give it a few years…

Since we've been back home, though, she's become a bit quiet. It will be an early night for her, and I'll see how she is in the morning. I had wondered about asking Mum or Karen to come and sit with her so I can go into work, but I'll just hang on. Besides, Mum has own things to worry about.

"How's Dad?" I ask.

"Oh, you know… he's *alright*," she says dubiously, making me think he is anything but.

"Mum…"

"Sorry, Alice. I don't want to trouble you with this, you have enough going on."

"Mum!" I say more sharply. "You won't be troubling me. What did the doctor say?"

"It wasn't so much the doctor as Phil himself, to be honest. What he had to say. I don't think I'd realised things had become so bad. I don't think he wanted me to. But he's not doing well. I mean, I don't think it's anything sinister, as they say, in that he's not about to keel over. But he's so worn out, Alice. And he's depressed, too. I think that was the bit that got me the most. Depressed and suffering from anxiety. Your dad's not the anxious type!"

My mind leaps back to the night Mum was in hospital, when Dad had been in a terrible state, but of course Mum wasn't there to witness that. I don't think that would be classed as anxiety, though, so much as a very natural reaction to a scary situation. She is right, that none of this is in Dad's nature. But illness and stress can do terrible things to a person.

"Where is he now?" I ask.

"He's out in the shed, having a tidy-up!" she laughs drily. "His usual way of coping with things – or maybe it's more correct to say not coping."

"Poor Dad."

"I know."

"Poor you, too," I remind her. "It's not easy living with somebody who's ill, and trying to keep on top of the business as well."

"Yes, well, that was the other thing I wanted to talk about."

"Oh yeah?"

43

"Yes, I know we touched on it the other day, but your father and I have decided we are definitely going to sell up."

"Really?" I had known it was coming, of course, and I realise that I have absolutely no right to feel this way about it, but the disappointment is evident in my voice.

"I'm sorry, love, I know how much it means to you."

"Don't be daft! That really doesn't matter. I haven't worked there for a long time, and you certainly can't keep it on just for my emotional connection with the place!"

"I'm quite attached to it too, you know," she reminds me gently.

"Of course you are. Of course. Sorry, Mum. But it's not the kind of business you can run forever. One of these days, Julie and I are going to find it too much running Amethi!" I smile and I'm happy to hear her laugh.

"You two will be there till your dying day!" she says. "You'll never leave."

"Well, that's a scary thought. But not one hundred per cent awful," I muse. "Anyway, you were saying… you're selling up. And are you planning to stay in Cornwall?" I ask, suddenly hit by the fear that they might want to up sticks altogether, and head back to the Midlands.

"Of course! Oh yes, love, there's no way we're leaving when you're here, and Sam and the kids. And we've made some lovely friends down here. I just think we need to accept we're not as young as we were. And to take our health seriously."

"I can't argue with that. The health bit, I mean."

"We were thinking maybe a bungalow, just round the coast a little way. If that doesn't make us sound too old. We want to be within walking distance of town – there's that lovely little stretch of coastal path, or else the road way, if the weather's awful – but I think we both feel like it would be nice to have a bit more space, and a bit more peace and quiet, especially in the summer months."

"Well, I can't say I blame you. That all sounds very sensible… and quite exciting! Looking for a new place!" I realise it's important to be positive about this, as it's not going to be easy for Mum and Dad. But I think they're absolutely right, and I hope that life will become easier for them once they've relinquished all the stress and strain of running the hotel. Although it will be sad to say goodbye to the Sail Loft, more than anything I am really glad that they are planning to stay round here.

"You're right! Don't tell your dad, but I've already been on Rightmove a few times. There are some lovely places. Not cheap, though."

"No, that's certainly true. But I think you'll find the right one for you."

"I hope so. Anyway, love, I just wanted to make sure you were the first person I told. I know you'll be busy with the kids now. If Holly's not feeling better tomorrow, let me know, and she can always come over here. She can lie around with your dad! I know you'll be needed at Amethi."

"Thank you, Mum!" How does she always know what I need? I hope that my kids wonder that about me when they're older.

"Also, Alice, don't mention this to anyone yet will you, please? We need to talk to Bea."

"Of course I won't. You take it easy tonight, and tell Dad to as well! I'll give you a ring in the morning. Love you."

"I love you too, Alice."

6

Mum is not the only one to ring with news. After I've put the kids to bed – Holly fell asleep about three pages into her story – I have just sat down in the lounge when my phone starts buzzing. Sam picks it up and glances at the screen. "David," he says, handing it to me.

"Hello stranger!" I answer with, because I know it will annoy David. He always says that things like that are a passive-aggressive way of saying somebody isn't pulling their weight in a friendship. However, I realise immediately that he is not in the mood for joking.

"Alice," he says, "I'm so relieved you're there."

"Is everyone OK?" I ask.

"Yeah, yeah, we're all OK," he says impatiently, "well, sort of."

My stomach drops with a jolt. Is he ill? Is Martin?

"It's Tyler," he says. "Well, it begins with Tyler, shall we say?"

"More school problems?" Tyler has been having some issues at his new school. At primary, the kids he grew up with just accepted that he's got two dads. At secondary, however, he's come up against some less pleasant children, who seem to have a problem with the fact that Tyler is adopted – and not just adopted, but by two gay men. It makes my blood boil when I think about it.

I take the phone into the hallway so that I can give David my full attention. Sitting on the next-to-bottom stair, my eyes are drawn to a scrape of mud on the skirting board, which I have definitely noticed before and meant to do something about.

"Yes, that same kid," David says grimly. "Only this time I've got myself in a bit of a mess."

"You've...? What's happened?"

David's answer is muffled.

"Sorry, David, I didn't catch that."

"I said, I punched the kid's dad."

I laugh out loud. I can't help it. David is not the punching sort. Not because he's gay. Just because he's not.

"It's not funny!" he protests, although I am sure I can hear a hint of amusement in his voice.

"Are you sure?"

"Yes, well, no. I mean... no, it's not funny. Punching somebody is never the answer."

"That sounds like something the headmaster's told you."

"It is!" he exclaims. "That's exactly what he said, to me, in front of Tyler, and this little... *kid*... who's been giving Ty a hard time, and this kid's dad, too."

"Oh David."

"I know. But that's not the worst of it."

"Oh no." I feel like I know what's coming.

"He wants to press charges."

"The head?"

"The dad."

"Oh. Shit. Did they call the police?"

47

"No, but he's threatening to. And you can imagine how that's going to go down at work. I think I'm finished, Alice. They're already looking for heads to chop. I've just given them the perfect excuse to use mine."

"But you've been there ages."

"So has everyone else. Honestly, I'm not special."

"You are to me," I chance a little light-heartedness.

"Well, you're just a bit odd anyway." Despite everything, David finds it hard to be a hundred per cent serious. "Alice…" he says, in lowered tones, "I can't believe I punched him! He was being such an arrogant bastard, though. And pretending his son wasn't an utter pain in the arse. Then he called me a… a… gaylord."

"Oh my god, has he stepped right out of the 1980s?"

"He certainly looks like it."

"And that was enough to make you see red?"

"It was the straw that broke the camel's back. Martin's not impressed," he whispers.

I can imagine. Martin is as straight-down-the-line as they come.

"But Alice, are you proud of me?"

"Do you know what, David? I am."

We hang up and, although I know it's not a very responsible reaction, I can't help but smile at this story, and at David's slightly misplaced pride – but I am genuinely proud of him, for standing up for himself and his son.

I go back into the lounge, flopping onto the settee next to Sam.

"Everything OK?" he asks.

"Erm… sort of. Not really. I mean, David punched someone."

48

"What?"

"I know. Not exactly in character for him, is it? But it was to do with the boy who's been bullying Tyler. David punched his dad!" Oh god. I'm grinning. And I'm meant to be a pacifist!

"Bloody hell," says Sam, admiringly.

"I know. He got pulled into the head's office."

"That's fairly embarrassing."

"Yeah, I don't think Martin's impressed. But David thinks the bloke's going to try and press charges."

"Oh no."

"Yep. That's not going to go down well at a law firm. I think David's quite worried. But I think he's also feeling pretty good about himself!"

"I'd do it, for either of our two," Sam says.

"Would you?" I can't imagine Sam hitting somebody any more than I can imagine David doing it.

He laughs. "I don't know, actually. But I guess if somebody's pissed you off enough, and you're protecting your kids, you'd do anything. Almost anything."

"You're right." I know I've become more confident in speaking up about things since I've had Ben and Holly. They are too young to do it for themselves, so I suppose it's my job to advocate on their behalf. This has nearly led to some spats in soft-play places, and other parenting arenas, but I haven't yet felt the need to punch anybody.

Sam puts his arm around me, and I sink back against him. On the armchair across from us, Meg grumbles in her sleep. "Maybe that other bloke will change his mind once he's calmed down a bit."

"I don't know. We've both just said what we'd do to protect our kids. He probably feels exactly the same, even if he's a homophobic idiot. Presumably this boy's getting his views from somewhere. I think David might be right to be worried."

7

In the morning, Holly is still not quite herself, although she has more colour in her cheeks, and I'm happy to see that she gobbles up her breakfast, washing it down with two glasses of orange juice. When it comes to getting dressed and when I suggest nursery, however, she starts to get stressed and tearful, and kicks off in a way I've never seen before. I thought I'd escaped the 'terrible twos' with her. Maybe now she's four it's payback time. Her face goes red with rage, and she doesn't want to wear anything I suggest, plucking irritably at her favourite jumper when I manage to get it on her. I don't know what to do. I don't want to push things and, while she may just be being a stubborn beast, I can see she's not herself really. I wish that I could just stay here with her, but I also have to get Ben to school, as Sam's had an early start today and already left the house. Somehow, I've got to make sure Ben's ready, and that Holly is OK. I think of Mum. She's got a lot on her plate too, but I know she wouldn't have offered to have Holly if she didn't mean it.

"Hi, love. Holly still poorly?"

"Yeah, well, she's not quite right. And she really doesn't want to go to nursery. Is it still OK for me to drop her with you?"

"Of course it is! Or I can come and get her."

"No, that's OK, I'll take Ben to school, then bring her to you. Thank you, Mum. I don't know what I'd do without you."

It's true. I really don't know what I would do without her, or Dad. I am so grateful that they moved down here. And so glad that they want to stay. The more I contemplate them taking life a little easier, the more I see it's the right thing for them to do. Dad will still be involved with the local council, and I know that will keep him busy, but hopefully not too busy. Mum… well, I don't know yet what she'll do. She won't be content doing nothing. I vaguely imagine her becoming more involved with Amethi. I imagine a job share between the two of us, and me being able to spend more time with Ben and Holly. Making the most of these last few months before Holly starts school, and being there for them when they get home. My inner feminist groans, but it's not about being a woman. It's just about wanting to spend time with my children. And worrying that I'm not always there for them when they need me. *Do you think Sam feels like this?* That little needling voice asks. *It's always the mums.* It doesn't matter, though, what other people think or do. This is my relationship with my children, and I really want to make sure that I get it right.

"OK," I tell Holly, kissing the top of her head. "You can go to Granny and Grandad's today."

"I want to go to the Sail Loft!" Ben shouts. "It's not fair!"

"I know, Ben." I go through to his room. "Me too. I've got to go to work, though. Tell you what, shall we see if you can have a sleepover there at the weekend?"

"Just me?" he asks.

"Just you," I smile.

"Yes!" He punches the air. As well as he and Holly get on with each other, it doesn't do any harm for them to have some one-on-one time with parents or grandparents.

"Come on now, though," I say, checking my watch. "Let's make sure we've got everything, and get on our way."

"OK, Mummy," Ben says, and I feel my heart melt a little. I pull him to me for a hug, and I feel a little tug on the back of my trousers. I turn to see Holly with a bag stuffed full of toys.

"You're ready too, are you?" I ask, and I pick her up, my other arm still around Ben. I take a moment, or two, just to hold them and feel them, soft and warm and solid in my arms. Ben's breath smells of toothpaste and Holly's smells of something sweet that I can't quite place. Damn, I've forgotten to brush her teeth. I think we're going to have to give it a miss this morning, though. We really need to go.

Holly insists on me carrying her from the car to the school gates, although I put her on the ground when we get there. "You'll be coming here in September," I tell her. "You want the teachers to see what a big girl you are, don't you?" I half hate myself for that. Who cares what people think? She's not feeling well. But it's a relief to my arms, and my back, for a while. Ben finds his friends immediately, and barely looks back when the teacher opens the door for them. Nevertheless, I stay to watch him go in, ignoring the little internal squeeze I feel as he disappears through the door into his own little world of school and friends and teachers. I stop for a brief chat with Sarah, who I met when Ben was a baby and whose twin boys are at this school too, before swinging Holly into the air and trotting with her back to the car, bumping her up and down so she laughs.

She's excited to get to the Sail Loft. We climb the stone steps to the front door, then Holly goes to the desk and rings the bell, as she always does. Mum steps out of the kitchen, mock-surprised to see us, and Holly runs into her arms.

I put the bag of toys on the reception desk. "Thank you so much, Mum. I'm really sorry to just cut and run."

"Don't be daft. You get going. We'll be here when you get back! Won't we, Holly? Now, do you want to help Granny make some cakes?"

"Yes! Chocolate cakes?"

"We can do chocolate cakes, no problem!"

"Thanks, Mum," I say, feeling a bit gutted that I can't stay and make cakes as well. Just a tiny part of me wishing I was still a child, and had Mum looking after me – or my grandma, my dad's mum, as she would have had me when Mum was at work. I wouldn't mind being able to relinquish some of the responsibilities that come with being an adult – just for a little while.

As soon as I'm on the road up to Amethi, however, I find I'm able to screw my work mind into place. It's a beautiful day, for once, and it's a relief to see blue sky ahead of me, even with the puffs of clouds that are moving rapidly across it. When I pull into the car park, I go to the boot to release Meg, who has been sitting quietly and patiently throughout the school run and Sail Loft drop-off. As she scampers to the hedge to check out what new smells might have materialised overnight, I notice that the breeze has picked up, and is ruffling the leaves of the protective tree line. Then I think... leaves! At last! It seems to have been a long time since those trees have looked anything other than bare – and an age since they've made any sound other than slightly disconcerting creaking when the wind's been blowing. I look up and see that yes, slowly but surely, there is a little carpet of green beginning to creep across the branches and down the finger-like offshoots. The jackdaws rise up almost as one, as though reacting to my scrutiny. I can't help but smile to think that maybe, just maybe, spring is about to make its presence known.

Lizzie is in the courtyard, pushing little bedding plants into the pots outside her front door.

"I'll miss seeing you here," I say.

"Alice. I will miss you, too. And you, Meg," she smiles as Meg runs up to greet her, pushing her nose firmly into Lizzie's hand. "I'm going to really enjoy this last summer here, though."

"And it's exciting," I say, not wanting to sound like I'm trying to make Lizzie feel bad.

"I think so," she says. "I mean... van life! Brilliant! But sharing with somebody else... it's a small space. And I've lived on my own for a long, long time."

Is it my imagination or is there a note of doubt in her voice?

"Yes, you have," I say, "and yes, a van is an extremely small space! But it's just a way to get to bigger spaces, isn't it? I can just see you and Med camping out under the stars, sleeping under an obelisk..."

"God, I hope not, they're really heavy!"

"You know what I mean!"

"I do. I suppose, it's a big step for me. It's… not quite a commitment, but it's sending a definite message.'

"Ah, but you and Med think the same way, don't you? And Lizzie, if for any reason it doesn't work out, we'll still be here. Me and Julie and Amethi."

Lizzie looks like she might be about to cry when I say this. That would be quite out of character for her. But when she speaks it's one of her slightly baffling and vague sentences, which I once found annoying but now consider endearing. "When change is coming, there's not much we can do to get in its way."

"But we all make our own choices," I counter.

"Yes, well, that's true. But sometimes they're not our choices to make."

I haven't heard Lizzie talk like this for a while. I guess she's unsettled about things. Putting my hand on her shoulder, I try to reassure her. "I mean it, Lizzie. Any time you want or need to come back, we're here. We are not going anywhere."

She just smiles.

Meg has trotted off somewhere, so I leave Lizzie to her planting, and I walk alone across the gravel, taking my time and listening to the birds singing. I can hear a buzzard somewhere distant but when I look up and scan the sky, I see no sign of it.

Unlocking the door to the office, I spring up the stairs, suddenly energised by the change in the weather. I unpack my laptop and charger and plug them in then I open the office window, even though it's not the warmest of days, just to feel like I'm still a part of the outside world, and to let a little of that blue-sky brightness in. Then I get to work. I have much to catch up with after yesterday. Coffee can wait.

It's lunchtime before I take a break, and I decide to eat outside. I may even uncover one of the tables and benches, in a burst of optimism. I make a single cafetière of coffee and slice off a thick wedge of wholemeal loaf, then scoop some houmous onto my plate. I add some roasted vegetables, slick and shiny with olive oil, and a few toasted pine nuts, then I carry the whole lot outside. I have just taken a bite of bread when my phone goes. I sigh and check the screen. It's Lydia.

"Hello there!" I say, trying to chew rapidly, grateful it's not a video call. "How's life in the media spotlight?"

She has been dating Si Davey, an increasingly famous and popular British actor, for some time now. He's a nice bloke, as I'd hope for Lydia, but I know she's finding there is a downside to her relationship. More than one – but the main problem being the lack of privacy. I recall some newspaper headlines when they went on their first holiday together, and nobody knew who Lydia was. Since then, her identity as the manager of the Bay Hotel has been uncovered, and more than once she has had 'guests' staying at the Bay who have turned out to be members of the British press, looking to dig up some dirt. They won't really find much on Lydia. I've known her since she was a teenager, waitressing at the Sail Loft when I was manager there. She went out with Jonathan, our then-chef, for quite a while, then went to uni and work in London. I can't vouch for what she got up to there, but she must have worked hard, because she's done very well for herself.

"It's nice to speak to somebody normal," she says.

"Boring, you mean?"

"Nope… normal! Not some up-themselves actor or actress."

"Ah yes, your weekend away! I'd forgotten! How was it?"

"Ermmm… I've had better."

She's been with Si and some of the cast of the TV programme he's been starring in.

"Oh no. Was it as bad as you'd anticipated?"

"Worse! Some of them are OK, but there are a couple of the cast who are so incredibly boring… and yet have no awareness of that fact − or of anyone around them. Si says they've done too much cocaine. Apparently, that's what happens; people assume that everyone else is really, really interested in everything they've got to say. Most of which is about themselves."

I laugh. "But it was a nice hotel?"

"Oh yeah, lovely! In fact, I spent more time chatting to the staff there and swapping notes than I spent with Si's mates… Actually, it's not really fair to call them mates. They're colleagues, really. But there's a sort of expectation of being sociable, and everyone getting on brilliantly well. It all feels a bit forced and uncomfortable."

"That's work for you!"

"I know, but not always. Look at you and Julie. You work together. You're practically married to each other."

"Ah yes, but we actively chose to work together. Our friendship came first. You all get on OK at the Bay, don't you?"

"Yes... mostly!" She goes quiet for a moment. "Si wants me to leave, though."

"Does he?"

"Yes. He's—" she breaks off and I imagine her looking around surreptitiously, to make sure nobody can hear – "been offered a part in an American film."

"Oh wow." I know I can't ask which film, or for any more details at all, in fact.

"I know. It is amazing. But..."

"You don't want to go?"

"I don't know. Not really. It will be riding on his coat-tails, won't it? You know that's not me, Alice."

"It's not, I know."

"But he'll be gone for months. Maybe a year. Maybe more."

"What would you do out there?"

"I have no idea. Get a job? But I won't know anyone. And I'll just be Si's girlfriend. And I've worked so hard at the Bay, to get it to what it is now."

"I know you have. Oh blimey, I wish I could tell you what's the right thing to do."

"I wish you could, too. I have no idea. And then on top of all this shit, there's Xavier."

"Oh, is that the agent? Is he still annoying?"

"Annoying doesn't cover it. It's so obvious he doesn't think I'm the right *calibre* for Si. I've a good mind to go to the States with Si just to piss Xavier off!"

"Tell you what, shall we meet up one evening soon, and have a proper chat about it all?" I do want to hear more, but I also want to eat my lunch.

"I was going to suggest that! Maybe you can come to me, though, just to make sure nobody's listening who shouldn't be. There is something else I want to talk to you about."

"That sounds interesting! Of course, I'll come to you." What a nightmare it must be, having to think through every little thing. I remember how many actors and musicians I had crushes on when I was growing up, and how I'd dreamed of being in a relationship with them. The reality is far from the fairy-tale I'd imagined back then. I'm very glad I'm with Sam. I wonder what this other thing is… Could she be pregnant? No, that doesn't really fit in with what she's saying about going to the US. It's probably something work-related.

Lydia and I check our diaries and manage to find a date we can both do. Then we hang up and I take a sip of my coffee, then a mouthful of houmous and vegetables, only for my phone to start buzzing again. Shall I ignore it? I check the screen and see that this time it's David. I'm going to have to take it. I can feel my lunchtime slipping away…

"They've made me redundant." David's voice is flat and despondent.

"What? Who?" I already know that's a stupid question. David is kind enough not to take issue with it.

"Work. I had to tell them about the… incident… before they found out some other way. I thought it would be better to be honest about things."

"Is he really going ahead with pressing charges, then?"

"I don't know, but I couldn't let it hang over my head like that." All traces of false pride at his actions have left David.

In the aftermath of the 'incident', I can imagine it felt amazing – he stood up for his son, and for himself and Martin. Perhaps that punch had the pent-up power of years of slights and snide comments, sometimes outright disgust, behind it. That one man took the brunt of all the frustration and anger that David has had to endure in the course of his life.

"Oh David," I say. "I'm sorry."

"I know. Thank you. It can't be helped. I shouldn't have acted like a meathead."

"I don't know if I'd quite put you in that category," I say.

"Well, you're in the minority," David says, and I'm pleased to detect he's smiling when he says this.

"So what happened? What did they say? At work, I mean."

"I just went in this morning and asked to see Barney, and Samantha from HR. I told them straight out what had happened, and in fairness they were very sympathetic, but their official line is that they can't have somebody working for them with a possible criminal charge coming their way. I get it. I knew what they'd have to do. And they've been looking to make redundancies anyway. If I'm honest, it was a slightly calculated move on my part. If I hadn't told them and then I'm charged with whatever, they'd have to sack me. By getting in first, I was able to explain things and they told me that I could take a redundancy package, if I wanted to. Otherwise, they'd have to discuss their options. Which probably means they'd end up giving me the shove anyway."

I take a moment to let this sink in. "So when do you leave?"

"I already have."

"Really?"

"Well, there's no point hanging around now. I've agreed to do a full handover of everything I've been working on, which I need to supply to Samantha, and that can all be divvied out between my esteemed colleagues. Divvy being the operative word."

At least he's still cracking jokes. "What did Martin say?"

"I haven't had a chance to tell him yet. He wasn't sure I should be saying anything, unless I actually had to, but I just couldn't fight this feeling that I needed to tell them."

"I get it. It would be really hard going into work every day, knowing that you were keeping this back from them."

"Exactly. I don't think I'd be able to focus, really. And... I don't know... they've been pretty good to me, letting me take that sabbatical to go to the US, and then letting me come back after the unexpected extension."

When covid struck, David and Martin stayed on in the States longer than they had planned to. They'd originally gone out to be near Bea, but then Bob died, and they couldn't leave Bea out there on her own. Now, thankfully, Bea and David are both back in Cornwall. Which is exactly where they belong, I think – only I wish it hadn't taken Bob's death to bring them home.

"They have been pretty good," I agree. "So... where are you now?"

"At home," he says glumly.

"And is Martin back tonight?"

"Yes, thank god, although not till late. I'll try and call him again in a bit."

"Alright. I'm up at Amethi, so just come up here if you want some company, or a bit of a wander in the woods.

Might be good to clear your head. And you won't bump into anyone you know up here."

"Thank you, Alice. I feel better for talking to you. I knew I would."

Throughout the afternoon, my mind flits between David and Lydia. David messages to say he's staying at home to work on his handover, and I decide that I'll take my advice to him if he's not going to, and head outside for a little wander in the woods. It's just a small patch of woodland, but it is full of life. Enveloped by birdsong, I stop for a while in the hide and my eyes become accustomed to the darker quality of light, and begin to pick out the movement between the trees and high up in the branches, of birds big and small flitting and darting busily about. There is a woodpecker somewhere up there, drilling away industriously, although I cannot see where exactly it is. And at the very top I can hear the jackdaws, cawing away, lording it over the smaller birds down below.

I think of the owls that we hear at night here. It's not often that I am here after six these days, and I remember with fondness my time living up at Amethi. I do love where we are now, and the suburban nature of our house and street hold their own comforts, but I miss this wilder, secluded world.

This is what Si and Lydia could do with, I think. A place where they can hide away, and just get on with life. But why should they have to hide anywhere? It's just stupid, really, the way certain individuals are targeted, as if they're any different to any other human being.

Sam's mum is one for reading those celeb magazines, when she's in the doctors' waiting room, or the hairdressers. She won't spend money on them, but she once reported back to me on a story about Si and an actress he was working with – insinuating there was something going on between them. "People want to read about all that stuff. They like the glamour of that world, Alice," Karen said, when I tutted at the story. "And those magazines are just feeding off that want. If people weren't interested, there would be no market for them."

"Well, yes, but also those magazines are just feeding that side of people. If they didn't exist, then nobody would be any the wiser." I already knew about the story Karen was referring to, as Lydia had told me all about it. She was sure there was nothing in it, and in fact Si has told her that the actress in question is a lesbian. But once something is in print, people latch onto it. "I suppose it brightens up boring lives," I suggest.

"Don't be so condescending, Alice!" Karen had said. "It's just a bit of fun, isn't it?"

"Not if you're the people being gossiped about," I bristled, not happy to be called condescending. But maybe she was right. I suppose I am looking down at people who like that kind of thing. It's just that it seems to overlook the fact that the subjects of their speculation are real people. Maybe they are financially richer than any of us could ever dream of being – and far better looking, too – but is that really a reason to pull their lives to pieces, and potentially damage their relationships? I don't suppose I really gave it that much thought before but now I know somebody who is affected directly, it bothers me. Lydia's stuck with this question of whether or not to go to the States with Si. What if she stays put? Will it be the end of things for the two of them? But what if she goes? What will that mean for her career – and her reputation?

David, meanwhile, knows that his own work is scuppered. I don't think he and Martin will be in any trouble financially but even so, it's a huge change to have to deal with. I can't help feeling grateful that my life is so settled. It hasn't always been, and no doubt there will be more challenges to come, but right now, I am grateful for some respite.

8

"How's she been?" I ask Mum, as Holly attaches herself to me limpet-like, her arms around my neck and legs around my waist.

"Oh, up and down," Mum says. "I think she just needs a rest. So Granny ended up making the cakes, didn't she?" Holly's head nods against my neck.

"Shall we give Mummy a cake? And send some home for Daddy and Ben as well?"

Holly nods again. "And Holly," I hear, from somewhere under my chin.

"And Holly!" Mum laughs. "But save it for after your tea, OK?"

"OK."

Mum packages up some cupcakes and I swear my stomach rumbles at the sight of them. I clutch the cakes in one hand, while still supporting Holly, and I go out to the car, fastening her into her seat.

"How are you feeling?" I ask, putting my hand to her forehead. I'm pleased she has not got a temperature.

"Tired," she says.

"Alright, well let's get home and have tea and a bath, and we can read more of your book. Maybe you'll feel better after a good night's sleep."

Only she doesn't want her tea. Ben sits and eats his beautifully, but Holly wriggles around on her chair and barely touches her pasta. Predictably, though, she still wants her cake.

"Go on, then," I say, and turn to Ben, pre-empting his protest: "It's just because she's poorly, OK? And I'd rather she eats something. When you're poorly, you get to eat what you feel like as well, don't you?"

He has no argument for this, and instead tucks into his cake with relish. I'm pleased that Holly manages to eat all of hers, and also that Sam arrives just as I'm clearing away their plates. It means he can give Ben some attention while I bath Holly. I still have that niggly guilty feeling that I haven't been with her while she's poorly, although I also have a similarly guilty feeling that I'm focusing on her more than on Ben so that I'm not giving him enough attention.

"I'll read to you after Holly's gone to sleep. Is that OK, Ben? We can have some proper time together then."

He's already busy looking at his Lego magazine with Sam, and I have to concede that I'm more bothered about these things than Ben seems to be.

Holly starts to get crotchety when we're upstairs and I'm running the bath. She's pulling at her clothes half-heartedly, and asking for a drink.

"In a minute," I say, not wanting to leave her alone with a half-full bath. I've never forgotten that line about it being possible to drown in an inch of water.

"I'm thirsty!" she exclaims, and she's close to tears. This is not looking good for her going back to nursery tomorrow, I think, contemplating how that knocks on to my work plans, and at the same time kicking myself for being so selfish.

"Right. Stay here. Do not get into the bath, I will be right back with some water for you, OK?"

"Milk!" she says.

"Milk's no good if you're thirsty. I'll get some squash," I compromise, and I dash down the stairs, disturbing Meg, who is lying at the front door, and who looks at me with mild interest before putting her head back down on her paws and sighing.

"Just getting Holly a drink!" I call through to Sam and Ben, although they haven't asked, and I am in and out of the kitchen in a flash, rushing back upstairs with all sorts of images in my head, but to my relief Holly is still sitting just where I left her, on the bathroom floor. She looks worn out, the poor little thing.

"Here you go, lovely girl," I say, handing her the cup, and she downs the drink in one go. "You really were thirsty. Come on, let's get you out of those clothes and into the bath. Just a quick one, and then we can get you into bed."

I marvel at her little body as I help her strip off, and swing her gently into the bath. This does at least make her giggle, I'm pleased to note. I check her surreptitiously for any signs of a rash, but I'm glad to see her skin is clear. Her little ribs are quite prominent, I notice. She's never been blessed with a lot of spare flesh, but she's definitely growing upwards rather than out. Ben's quite tall for his age, and I think she will be the same.

I don't bother washing her hair, but just help her soap herself and rinse off, then I wrap her up in a nice clean towel and bump her gently up and down on my knees while I dry her, as I know she loves it when I do that. Her head rests gently against me and she protests at the thought of doing her teeth, but I insist, and then it's off to bed with her.

I'm fully expecting her to fall asleep within minutes, but instead she is restless, and she says she needs a wee, then she says she needs a drink. My mind is starting to turn towards Ben, downstairs, and my promise to read to him at bedtime. I push back any thoughts to do with work, and what I will do if Holly's still ill tomorrow. I will deal with that if it comes to it.

"Come on, Holly," I say gently. "Just put your head down, and get some sleep."

"I need a drink," she protests, and luckily Sam pops his head in at that moment.

"Can you get her some water please?" I ask.

"Of course. Shall I send Ben up, too?"

"Yes, tell him I'll be with him in a few minutes," I say, optimistically.

I look back at Holly and I'm relieved to see her eyelids fluttering. It takes me back to her baby days, and Ben's, when I sometimes would sit with them while they drifted off into their little dreamworlds; watching their eyes roll back slightly disconcertingly as delicate lids flicked down then up again, then down for a longer time, until they could fight sleep no more.

By the time Sam has returned, complete with a bottle of water, Holly is snoring gently. I stroke her forehead and sit for just another couple of minutes before making an exit and going to find Ben. He is minty-fresh and waiting in his bed, a Mr Gum book in his hands. I'm glad. I love these books at least as much as he does. I cave into his demands for two extra chapters, wanting to make up for the lack of time I've had with him today, then I hold his hand while he goes to sleep. Thankfully, it doesn't take long, and I tiptoe down the stairs to Sam. I sink gratefully onto the settee. A slice of late evening sunshine falls through the window onto us; it reminds me that summer is on its way and I am so glad. I always have more energy during those months. I lean against Sam with my eyes on the television but my thoughts on Amethi, and the mounting bills, and Lizzie leaving, and Holly being ill, and Dad being ill, and Luke being depressed, and David losing his job, and...

"You're tensing up," Sam says, looking at me.

"Am I?"

"Yes! Are you worried about Holly?"

"Amongst other things," I say.

"She'll be alright. Kids bounce back, don't they?" Sam says, reassuringly.

"Yes, they do," I agree but while I know that he's right, I feel uncomfortable. "I might just take Meg out for a walk," I say. "If you don't mind."

"Of course not. It's a good idea."

"Maybe even down to the beach. I might hop in the car, though," I say, semi-apologetically. I don't like taking the car for unnecessary short journeys.

"Why don't you go for a swim instead? You should see if Julie wants to join you."

"Do you know what? That is a great idea. We must have another hour or so of light left in the day." My spirits lift at the thought, and within minutes I've called Julie.

"That is a brilliant idea," she says. "I was hoping to catch up with you one evening this week. There's something I need to talk to you about.'

I hope she's not going to ask about having an anniversary party. That would be just typical. I suppose in that case I might have to tell her my plans. A little part of me likes the idea of no longer having to keep such a secret. Anyway, I'll see what she has to say. Lydia also crosses my mind and I wonder idly what's going on with her.

Within minutes, I've changed into my swimming things, and I'm on my way to pick my friend up, heading for some much-needed moments of abandon in the cold, fresh saltwater of this beautiful bay.

9

"Ahhhhhhhh…" I sigh, once I've acclimatised to the cold water wrapping itself around me. I like to take my time easing myself into the waves, splashing a bit of the shocking cold onto my shoulders, the tops of my arms, my neck… trying to convince my body that this is all perfectly normal.

Julie, on the other hand, practically sprinted in, shouting into the sky as she went. It definitely feels like she needs some sense of abandon, putting dry land and the realities of life behind her, if only for a little while.

Now we have met on an even keel, floating on our backs, necks cricked slightly so we can see and talk to each other, sculling with our hands while the incoming waves lift and lower us gently as they pass below before breaking a couple of metres in towards shore.

"How's Holly?" Julie asks, at exactly the same time that I say, "How's Luke?"

"You first," she says, and I accept without argument, sensing she perhaps does not want to talk about Luke just yet.

"Oh, I don't know," I say. "I thought she seemed a bit better earlier, but she was really worn out by bedtime."

"Hopefully that means she'll sleep," Julie suggests.

"Let's hope so." I can't quite quell the feeling of unease

about my little girl, but I guess it's normal. I had never fully appreciated the pressure of responsibility that comes with being a parent. I've had the guilt when I've sent Ben into school complaining of a tummy-ache, only for them to ring me an hour later and say he'd been sick in the classroom. In fact, guilt features heavily in the whole parenting experience, as far as I can tell. I try to suppress it now, thinking here I am floating on the waves with Julie while Holly's poorly in bed.

"You need this," Julie says, as though she can hear my unspoken thoughts. "To be able to go back and do your job properly, as a mum, I mean. You have to have some time out to refresh yourself and get your energy levels back up."

"I know you're right. And you too. It looked like you'd never stop running, the way you were charging into the sea!"

"Yeah… well…"

"Luke still bad? Not bad… You know what I mean." I feel my hair swirling around my shoulders in the water, and the sun breaks free of a cloud, sending a shaft of warmth across us. Before long, though, night will start to fall. The thought sends a little shiver through me.

"I do know!" She smiles. "And he is actually doing a bit better, thanks, Alice. A bit more like himself. He's drinking less, too."

"Well, that's good." There is a slight question in my voice. I can sense that she's not telling me everything.

"Yes… it is. Of course it is. But, Alice…"

"What?" I ask, swivelling my body so that now I'm upright and treading water. Julie does the same, so we're facing each other, and I see that there are tears in her eyes.

"I don't know how to tell you this."

73

"What?" I ask, my mind leaping ahead to all sorts of possible, awful conclusions.

"I think we're..." she stops, changes tack – she is a big believer in being direct. "We are planning to leave Cornwall." Her eyes seek out mine and scan my face for reaction. But I don't seem to be able to summon one immediately.

"You're...?"

"Leaving Cornwall," she says.

"But... how...? Where?" I am stuttering, trying to process what Julie has just said. This can't be right, can it?

"We're thinking of going abroad. Canada, maybe. A city. Toronto seems good."

"Toronto seems good?" I exclaim.

"Yes. It's... there's a lot going on. And there are a lot of different people there. You know – racially, for a start."

"But you haven't had any problems here," I say. "Or Zinnia... has she?"

"No, not at all. And that really is just a small part of it. God, this is difficult," she says.

"You're telling me." I look out to the horizon, tears biting at my eyes and a lump rising in my throat. I want to swim, far out, and just keep swimming. Instead, I turn, and start heading back to shore, with strong, firm strokes.

"Alice!" I hear Julie behind me, but I keep going, and I walk out of the sea back towards our towels, goose pimples prickling the full length of me. I'm shivering, and shaking, and I don't know if it's the effect of the cold water, emerging into the cold air, or the shock of Julie's announcement.

I begin drying myself off and Julie stands next to me, her wet skin and hair glistening in the late sunshine.

"Alice!" she says again. "I'm sorry."

"It's fine."

"No. It's not fine. It's far from fine. It's been eating away at me, all this. I'm torn. I really am. But it's got to be family first," she says softly.

"I thought we were family," I say, and I hear the childish petulance in my voice.

"Yes. But... Luke's my husband. And Zinnia's my daughter. And you've got Sam, and Ben, and Holly... They're your priority. Luke and Zinnia are mine."

"What about Amethi?" I ask quietly. When Julie and Luke went to India, we had to find a way to manage without her input as a chef, but we knew it was just temporary. This news, this plan to leave for Toronto, has an air of permanence about it.

"I'm going to have to sell my part of it," she says, wrapping her towel around herself, then looking me in the eye. "I'm so sorry, Alice. We can't afford to do the same as before, and it wouldn't make sense, anyway. We want to start afresh somewhere. You'll have first refusal, of course, if you can raise the funds, but I know it's not as easy as that."

"But without you, it won't be Amethi. That place is you and me, Julie. You know that."

"I do," she says, sadly. "And I love it. But you know it's been draining both of us recently – financially, and energetically. I never thought about an ending for it when we took it on, but lately I've been thinking it can't go on forever. Not for me, anyway," she says apologetically. "We've had a decade there, and it has been amazing. But I think I want to do something different. I think maybe I want to work for somebody else for a bit. You know how hard it is, trying to cover all the increased costs. The responsibility! You know me and responsibility," she tries a small smile, to see if I'll reciprocate. I don't. She continues. "I know it's bothering you as well. And for us, with everything else that's happened, losing Jim… I want to relieve some of that pressure of owning a business. Or maybe Luke and I will start something together at some point. I don't know."

It hurts like hell. I feel a bit like I can't breathe, but I know that is incredibly melodramatic. I don't know what is worse – that she is planning to leave me, and Amethi, or that she's clearly been thinking and planning and discussing all the different options, without giving me so much as an inkling.

I start to shove my things into my bag, not looking at Julie. I can't. I want to run away and cry, which is just pathetic, but it's how I feel. Instead, I have to wait for her, and give her a lift home.

"Alice," Julie says, but I don't look up. "I mean… look out there, at the sea."

I turn my head and cast my eyes across the waves. In the last light of day, slipping and diving through the water, not all that far from where we just were, is a pod of dolphins. And yet, despite the magic of this sight, right now it barely makes me feel anything. I push a slight smile onto my face, and try to meet my friend's gaze, but it just doesn't want to happen. I can't fool anyone, least of all myself.

The car journey back is quiet and contemplative. Julie tries a couple of times to make conversation, but we know each other well enough to just leave it for now.

"I'll see you tomorrow," I say, when I pull up outside her house. "Honestly, I'm not pissed off with you, even though I know it seems like it. It's been an awful time for Luke and you. I get it. I just need to let it sink in. I need to think it all through."

"I know. I get it, too. And there is no rush. We're not about to just run off, and even when we do go, I won't necessarily need to sell up straight away."

"Just give me some time, Julie," I say, and I want to reach over, open the door for her, let her out. Away from me. For now.

She sees me glance at the door handle, and gets the message. "Alright," she says, and I hate to hear the dejection in her voice. "Maybe we can talk tomorrow."

"I'm sure," I say flatly. "See you tomorrow."

"Love you, Alice."

"Love you, too." Because I do. Of course I do. Otherwise I wouldn't care so much. I remember Luke saying at his mum's funeral, all those years ago, how we need to let people know how we feel about them while they are alive – meaning don't wait for a eulogy to say how you feel – and it has always stuck with me. Even now, my feelings in turmoil, I need Julie to know how I feel about her. Because she is my family, my sister, in every way that matters. And I will always love her.

Driving off towards home, I realise I am not quite ready to go back yet. Instead, I find myself driving up and out of town, and inland, to the top of the hill – a place called Carn Brea. A Neolithic settlement and fort, it's easy to see why this place was chosen, as the views from here are breathtaking for me but would have also been incredibly useful to those who settled here, to keep an eye out for any threat.

I need a torch to help me find my way carefully up the rocky path, and by the time I get to the top, where the ancient stones rest, dusk has sunk around me. In daylight, on a clear day, it is possible to see across towards all sides of this part of Cornwall, with tin mines and railway lines, the sea not far away. More modern additions to the industrial side of this landscape include a huge B&M store and Tesco, which sit alongside a range of other shops and a heritage centre. There is something about the sight of the lights spreading out around me and into the distance – shops and roads, cars, lorries, buses; houses, hotels, homes, which I find comforting. I hope it will help me find some balance, and straighten out my thoughts. I sit and I breathe slowly, holding my breath for a moment with each inhale, and then again at the end of each exhale.

A crew of ghostlike gulls forges their way overhead. I watch them vanish into the darkness and then I place my hands on the cool rocks, wondering who else has touched this very place over the ages. I breathe, and I think. Breathe, and think.

Julie is going. Amethi is over.

This was not how I imagined it. Because, of course, I hadn't thought it was absolutely forever. But I also had not ever contemplated the end, other than in the loosest possible fashion, idly imagining what might lie ahead. Far ahead. Always assuming it would be a conclusion that Julie and I reached together.

I dig deep, to try and fathom my feelings towards my

friend. I told her I am not pissed off with her, but am I? No, I find. Not really. Because it is her life. Hers and Luke's and Zinnia's. And Julie has always been a little more restless than me. Luke, too; he likes city life, and he loves travelling. And he's coming to terms with being, in effect, an orphan. Not in a maltreated Oliver Twist way, but a man without either parent. If anything can make you re-evaluate your life, surely that must. I think of his behaviour after Jim's funeral. He has been deeply, deeply unhappy, and that cannot carry on. If that means moving to Canada, so be it. But yet... all of this is at the expense of Amethi. And the expense of me, and my happiness. And Sam's. What will we do without Julie and Luke? And what will Ben and Holly do, without Zinnia? They will probably be OK. *Kids bounce back*, Sam said, and I know he was talking about illnesses, but they do adapt well; probably better than us, and better than we give them credit for. It is me and Sam who will suffer. But how much more would we suffer to see Luke sink into a deep depression, or alcoholism, or both?

I trudge disconsolately back down the path, taking each step tentatively as the darkness firmly closes its teeth around the very last of the daylight. Stopping for a moment, I look down once more at the lights of the towns and villages strewn across this beautiful land. There is life all around me, unaffected by what to me is disastrous news. There will be people out there having the time of their lives, and there will be people out there dealing with tragedies, disasters, stress. Throughout everything, life goes on.

I get back into the car, and turn around to head home. I will break the news to Sam, if Luke has not already done so, and then I will get an early night, and hope that a good sleep brings some perspective.

Except... I arrive home to find that Holly is awake, and attached to Sam like a little monkey. As soon as she sees me, she turns around and holds out her arms. "Mummy," she says, emitting a sob.

"Hey darling," I say, weighing up the situation in a moment, and taking her from Sam, all thoughts of Julie's news banished for the moment. Holly does not look well. "What's up?"

"She wet the bed," says Sam. "I've been trying to strip off all the wet stuff but it's hard to do that and hold her at the same time!"

I feel really bad that I took that bit of time for myself, going up to the carn, when I should have come straight home.

"I'll go and sort it all now," he says. "Maybe I should sleep in the spare room tonight, and she can go in with you? I think we're going to have to wash the mattress somehow, too."

Oh no. This is not good, and it is completely out of the blue, for Holly has never been a bed-wetter. Not that it would matter if she was, but after a few nights out of nappies we realised that there was no need for pull-ups, or, I thought, to put down waterproof sheets under her normal ones. Stupid, really. I guess it's inevitable kids will have accidents from time to time. I make a mental note to put one back on Ben's bed in the morning as well, just in case.

"Is Ben asleep?" I ask, rocking Holly back and forth.

"Yes, he's slept through everything, of course!" Sam grins, although I can see a strand of worry etched onto this forehead. "I don't think she's over her bug, though. And she's been drinking loads."

"That could be a good thing, help flush the germs out."

I follow Sam upstairs and gently put Holly down in the bathroom so she can go to the loo before going back to sleep. Then I gather her up and take her into our bed, where I tuck her in, then lie down on the covers next to her. My thoughts are swirling, and I feel like my heart's beating just a tad too fast. I need to slow down. I should go and help Sam, but I'm shattered, and don't think I will bother with a shower tonight. Instead, I rest my head against Holly's, and I hear her breathing begin to slow down, and breaths begin to lengthen, as she drops off to sleep. In time, my eyelids begin to droop too, and the next thing I know, Sam is tucking a blanket over me, kissing me on the head, and then kissing Holly, and turning the light off before creeping out of the room. He shuts the door softly, only now I'm wide awake again, Julie's shocking news hitting me afresh, alongside that growing feeling of unease about Holly.

I shut my eyes, desperate for some respite – only of course when you're thinking about sleep, it never comes. Without Sam by my side, I have nobody to talk to, and nobody to tell me that things will be OK. I listen to my little girl wriggle restlessly around, though she seems to be fast asleep, and I gradually accept that I'm in for a long, lonely night.

10

As if things weren't bad enough, at some point perhaps not too long after I had finally dropped off again, Holly had wet our bed, and she woke up crying and shivering, her pyjamas wet through. My mind a sleepy blur, I shook myself awake, and it took me a couple of moments to come up with a plan. I didn't want to wake Sam; much less Ben, so I stripped Holly and wrapped her in a throw, thinking she really needed a bath, but I couldn't let the bed situation get any worse. I made a little mattress for her with our pillows and instructed her to curl up on it, which she did without too much objection, and then I set to work pulling the duvet, sheet, and mattress protector from the bed, very grateful to see that Holly must have been tangled in the duvet and it had fared worst, while the mattress remained unscathed. I was able to bundle all the wet stuff onto the landing, but then I was stuck. All the clean bedding was in the spare room with Sam, and besides, what if Holly did the same thing again? My 2am brain decided the obvious thing would be to set up camp in the lounge, with our blow-up airbeds, so I dressed Holly in fresh pyjamas and carried her downstairs, plonking her on the settee and getting her the drink she was asking for, before digging out our camping gear from the depths of the garage, and blowing up the two single airbeds. I got Holly onto hers, as soon as I could, putting a waterproof sheet under the throw she'd been snuggling in, then putting a couple of open sleeping bags on top of her. I switched off the light, and wriggled into my sleeping bag, once more wide awake, but I must have been so tired that it didn't take too long for me to fall asleep.

I was woken this morning by Ben exclaiming at the sight of his mum and his sister camping out in the lounge. I was immediately wide awake, and I looked across to see Holly trying to keep her eyes screwed shut. She must have been exhausted after so much broken sleep, on top of not feeling one hundred per cent well.

"What's all this?" Sam asked, following Ben in. I could see he too was bemused, and also amused.

My first reaction was to put my hand across to Holly's bed, which thankfully was dry. It was enough for Sam to understand, though, and I saw a little cloud cross his face.

"Holly was feeling a bit thirsty, weren't you, sweetie, and so we came down here, and then we decided to camp out," I fabricated, not sure if she would want her brother to know the truth.

"I weed in Mummy's bed," she said.

That answered that question.

"Urgh! Did you?" Ben asked.

"Yes, she did. Holly's a little bit poorly, Ben. I might take her to the doctor this morning, I think." I directed this last line towards Sam.

"That's a good idea," he said. "You must be shattered, though. Maybe you and she can get a rest a bit later. I'll put the kettle on now, though. And get you sorted for school, young Benny!" He swung Ben into the air, and mock-groaned, holding his back. "You're getting too big for this kind of carry-on!"

"Are you hungry, Holly?" I asked, looking into her big blue eyes. She nodded.

"Come on, then. Let's get this day started," I say. "You go into the kitchen with Daddy and Ben, and I'll just sort this lot out."

"Can I sleep in the lounge tonight?" Ben called through.

"Erm… I don't see why not."

"Brilliant!"

"I might just go and have a shower," I told Sam, and I trudged up the stairs, feeling utterly shattered. I stepped gratefully under the hot water, allowing myself only a few minutes, as I knew I would need to be ready to get on the phone to the surgery as early as possible. Appointments are hard to come by these days, although if it's a child they will normally find a way to fit you in.

When I came back downstairs, my hair wrapped in a towel, I was glad to see Holly tucking into some Weetabix, while Ben informed me that he was on his second bowl.

"Really?" I asked, giving him a kiss on his head. "Well make sure you save some for me!"

While Sam was getting the kids dressed, I called the doctors, to be put into a queue, so I put the phone on speaker setting while I tidied up the mess. Just as I was wiping a spatter of mushy Weetabix and milk from the table, the receptionist answered.

"Hello!" I called, leaving the wet cloth on the table, and dashing to the phone. "Hi. I'm calling about my daughter."

"Can I take her name and date of birth please?"

I told her the details then explained what was happening with Holly. "I think it might be a urine infection," I said.

"What are her symptoms please?"

"Well she has wet the bed a couple of times, and keeps needing to go to the loo. She's really thirsty as well."

"OK. Let me see… could you get here for ten past nine?"

"Erm… yeah…" I looked at the kitchen clock. "Of course. Thank you." With a bit of luck, we'd get some antibiotics and start to kick this illness into touch.

"We've got an appointment," I called up to Sam. "I'll take Ben to school then we can go straight to the doctors from there."

"Are you sure you can do it? What about Amethi?"

"That's my next call," I said. "I'll ring Lizzie and see if she's about, to cover the phone."

"Can't Julie do it?"

"I don't know." I didn't want to think about Julie, and the bombshell she'd dropped on me last night. "It will be easier for Lizzie, she's already there. Then hopefully I can get in later and Julie can come in as normal. She'll be working late tonight, I think."

I didn't want to get into the Julie and Luke stuff at that point in the day, although I knew I'd have to tell Sam soon. One thing at a time, though. I had to get Ben to school, and Holly to the doctors. Both kids were beautifully well behaved, which made things a little bit easier, and Ben ran off into school happily. Tick. Next thing on the list: get Holly sorted.

"You say she's been wetting the bed?" the doctor asks. She is gazing at Holly thoughtfully, but she smiles when my daughter looks her way.

"Yes, just last night, a couple of times," I answer quickly. "But she never has before. Which is why I'm wondering if it's a water infection."

She seems to ignore my suggestion. "And is there anything upsetting her? Anything new, or different, at home, or nursery?"

"No," I said indignantly. "There's nothing upsetting her. At least... I don't think so." Doubt sets in. Is there anything upsetting her? New staff at nursery? New children? "No, I really don't think so," I say earnestly.

"Alright, that's fine. Perhaps I can just do a few checks, Holly, if that's OK?"

Holly nods.

"Can I listen to your chest?"

Holly obligingly lifts up her t-shirt, and the doctor listens, apologising for the cold stethoscope. She looks in Holly's ears, in her throat, and she asks Holly to breathe out. I can see she's thinking about something. "Holly," she says, "Do you think you'd be able to do a wee? Into a little container, if you take it to the toilet and Mummy helps you?" She looks at me. "Is that OK?"

"Of course," I say.

"Great, then if you can just take this with you into the toilet next door—" she hands me the container – "and come back when it's done, you can leave it in there and I'll do a couple of tests on it. Just to rule a few things out."

What few things? I want to ask. I never like the suggestion that things are being ruled out, as it always suggests to me that they are more likely being ruled in. Something stops me asking, and I obediently take the dish with me, holding Holly's hand and going into the toilet. It is all done in a moment, and I leave the bowl on the side, carrying Holly back into the doctor's room and sitting down with my daughter on my knee. The doctor is gone for a few minutes. When she comes back, I look at her expectantly.

"I might have to do another test," she says apologetically. She pulls a little black machine from a case and slides a slip of paper into it. "I'm sorry, Holly, I need to take a teeny tiny sample of your blood, from one of your fingers. Can you be very brave?"

Holly nods, and holds out her hand. "Ow!" she exclaims, as the doctor pricks the pad of her middle finger. Holly tries to pull her hand back, but the doctor holds it gently, while she puts the paper to the round, dark red drop of blood that sits on Holly's skin.

"What's this for?" I finally ask, but the doctor is watching the machine, which I see is counting down seconds. It gets to one, then a number appears. 19.1.

"What is that?" I ask.

"Mrs Branvall," the doctor says, looking me in the eye. "I'm really sorry but you're going to have to get Holly to hospital. It looks like she has type one diabetes."

From that point on, everything is a bit of a whirl. Keeping Holly calm is my priority, and making sure that she isn't scared, although to be honest none of this will mean much to her, while those words have hit me like a blow to the stomach.

"Are you sure?" I ask.

"Fairly," the doctor says. "Well, yes, really. I don't want to give you a load of flannel, Mrs Branvall. That is a very high blood glucose reading and I would think it is very unlikely that Holly's levels would be that high for any other reason."

"Could… could the machine be wrong?" What do I know about diabetes? I know it's serious. But lots of people have it, don't they? I recall a programme called *Children's Ward*, which I used to watch when I was a kid. There was a boy on that with diabetes – he stayed in my mind for some reason – and he had to have an injection at the start and end of each day, as I recall. Oh god. Injections. How is that going to go down with Holly? But then, I know other people – older people – who have diabetes and just have tablets, and I am sure I saw something about people reversing it with diet. A guest from my time at the Sail Loft springs to mind. That's going back a bit now. I remember her being quite ill with it.

Breathe, Lizzie's voice springs to mind. I'll have to tell her I won't be in till later, or maybe not at all, depending how long things take at the hospital.

"I doubt it, to be honest. I am really sorry," the doctor meets my gaze. "But lots of children have diabetes. More now than ever. And they live with it perfectly well. But it is important to get Holly seen today, because it could make her poorly if it's left untreated. As it is, you've done a great job getting her seen today. Because you seem very healthy and well to me, Holly. Am I right?"

Holly nods. I can't see her face, but I can imagine her

beaming. She certainly responds well to praise, does our girl.

"I'll call them now for you, if that's OK. It's the Royal Cornwall in Truro. Can you get there yourself?"

"Yes, yes, I think so," I say, feeling panic fluttering within me. "I must tell my husband. He'll need to get our son from school."

"Of course. Let me just speak to somebody at the hospital and find out what's what, then you can give him a ring. You'll probably need to ask him to bring you and Holly an overnight bag."

Overnight? This is not good. But maybe, as Holly is so well, it won't be necessary. I wait patiently, holding Holly to me and trying to breathe evenly, while we listen to one side of the phone conversation. "Yes… she's four and presenting with BG of 19.1… yes, with her mother. They can come straight away –" she looks to me for confirmation, and I nod – "that's great. Thank you."

"OK, Mrs Branvall. They're expecting you, if you can make your way straight to the children's ward… don't worry, I'll write this down for you. "They'll do a few more tests on Holly, just to confirm, or otherwise, and they'll take wonderful care of you there. Alright?" Her forehead is knitted with concern. I can feel tears in my eyes but I need to hold them back. I just nod.

"Thank you," I manage.

"Let me know how you get on, OK?"

"I will. Come on Holly," I say, conjuring up my cheerful, confident voice. "We need to get you to the hospital to go and see what's going on with you."

"In an ambulance?" Holly asks.

"No, Mummy will take you in the car," I say, to her evident disappointment.

"You're sure you're OK driving?" asks the doctor.

"Of course, yes, we'll be fine." I am already drawing on my inner reserves, to calm myself and keep things as normal as possible for Holly. "Thank you," I say again, and Holly and I walk hand-in-hand out of the surgery, the automatic doors opening to let us out into what might just be a very different world to the one that we left when we walked in.

11

At the hospital, it's hard to find a parking space, but there is a very tight one in a corner and I just go for it, slotting the car in as carefully as I can. Normally, I would drive around until I find a more spacious slot, but today it feels like there just is not time for that.

I've left a message for Sam, and I hope he'll be able to pick it up soon. If I don't hear from him by two, I'll call Mum, or Karen, because somebody will need to get Ben from school. I could ask Julie, of course, but it feels like something is blocking me from getting in touch today. I think I'm feeling angry at her. But I also know I am not thinking straight. I want to push all of that aside until I'm in a position to be able to really think about it sensibly.

I carry Holly across the car park, trotting along and making clip-clop noises, which makes her laugh. We go in through another set of automatic doors and see the signs to the children's ward.

Setting Holly on her feet when we get to the door, I use the hand sanitiser and press the intercom button. I tell them who we are, and we are buzzed through, then taken to the assessment ward. All the staff are very friendly, as you might expect. We are taken to a small room with a bed, where one of the nurses, who introduces herself as Angela, does a few tests on Holly, checking her weight, height blood pressure, etc., and we are soon joined by a woman with a kind face, and a stethoscope around her neck.

"Hello, Holly. I'm Dr Carter. I've just been hearing all about you from your doctor, and it's very nice to meet you in person. Have you been in hospital before?"

Holly shakes her head.

"Not even when she was born," I tell her. "We were stuck because of the snow."

"Sounds like you had a very dramatic entrance to the world!" Dr Carter laughs.

Holly is reluctant to give her hand over for another finger prick test, but she agrees to it. The doctor uses a similar machine to the one at the GP's and I see that the number this time is 17.7. So it's gone down.

"That's lower than earlier," I say hopefully.

Dr Carter smiles. "It's still very high," she says, adding quickly, "I've seen higher. You've done a very good thing, getting Holly in so quickly."

"So it is diabetes?" I ask dejectedly.

"It is," she says. "It must be."

"What should a normal reading be?"

"Well there's no one number, but ideally, it should be below 7."

"Oh. It is quite high, then."

"It is. We can keep an eye on it now you're here."

"So do we need to stay in overnight?"

"Yes, I would say so. Maybe more than one night."

"Really?" I can feel my face drop. I can't afford to spend time in hospital. But of course, I can't afford not to.

"Yes, it takes a bit of getting used to, learning how to do all the diabetes care. I won't go into it now. I promise it will be OK, and we will look after you and Holly so well. You will want to know that you can go out confidently into the world, though, both of you. And I'll be honest, I think as a mum you will need time to get your head round it and let it all sink in."

Angela lays a hand on my arm and that simple, kind touch brings tears springing to my eyes. "Look, let me go and see if they've got a bed ready, and I can take you and Holly through, OK?"

"OK." I nod. Holly turns to me, and I switch on my smile. She puts her arms around me and lays her head on my shoulder.

"Are you tired, Holly?" Dr Carter asks.

Holly just nods, against my neck. "Ahh, well we'll have a lovely bed for you, and you can have a nice rest, OK? Angela will go and see if it's ready. Now, I have to go and check on some other children, but I will be back to see you later, OK?"

She smiles at me, and I can see the sympathy in her eyes, then she and Angela leave, and it is just me and Holly, alone in the stark, clinical room. I hold my little girl close to me, and I allow myself a few silent, unseen tears. At the sound of the door being opened, I wipe them away with one hand. Angela has returned with a colleague. "Hello again, Holly!" She smiles brightly. "This is Chrissie, and she's going to show you and Mummy where you'll be sleeping tonight, OK?"

Holly nods. I stand up to carry her, and Chrissie smiles at me. She puts a guiding hand on my elbow. "Come on," she says. "You've got one of our private rooms."

"Your own private room, Holly!" exclaims Angela. "You'll have your own bathroom, your own TV. It's like being in a hotel!"

I smile at her. "Thank you."

"It's no problem. I'll come and see how you're doing later."

Chrissie is just as lovely as Angela. "This way," she says, walking us past the nurses' station in the centre of the ward, and leading us into a small private room. She pulls the blinds so we have privacy, and gestures for me to put Holly on the bed. She pulls up a chair so I can sit down next to her.

"Right," she says. "So this is where we are. Holly, you have something called type one diabetes. Do you know what that is?"

Holly shakes her head.

"I'm not surprised. Lots of people don't know about it, but we have lots of special girls and boys like you who come to us because they have type one. And the first thing that I need to tell you and your mum is that it is absolutely one hundred per cent not because of anything you've done, or not done. It's not because of eating sweets, or drinking fizzy drinks, and it's not because you don't do enough exercise. It is just because. OK?"

I know she is saying this more for my benefit than Holly's, and I do appreciate it, although I also wonder if she is saying it to make me feel better. I mean… diabetes… but I do really know that it is an illness that can come out of nowhere. I have known other people with it. I just hadn't expected my own child to have it.

"But it is something that isn't going to go away. And we are going to have to teach you and Mummy, and anyone else who needs to know, how to manage it. OK?"

Holly nods again.

"Great. Well, I can already tell you're going to be brilliant. Now if you want to settle in, I'm going to go away and get the diabetes kit, which has lots of clever little things in it, and some books for children, and for adults, and we will go through it all together. I'm afraid I will have to give you an injection very soon as well, to start making you feel better."

At that, Holly looks at me with fear in her eyes. It makes my heart clench. It's not all that long since she had her pre-school booster jabs, and that did not go well. But Chrissie is prepared for this.

"Now, it won't be like those injections you had at the doctors, OK? This is just a teeny-tiny needle, and you can look at Mummy when we do the first one, and you'll hardly even notice it, alright?"

I can see Holly isn't convinced.

She was right to be suspicious, as far as I can tell, from the amount of noise she makes. It takes every ounce of strength I have not to break down in front of her. I can't bear it. And we're going to have to do this not just twice a day, I learn, but multiple times – five, at least. And there are two types of insulin: one is a basal type that will last throughout the day and night, and one is for bolus injections, which she must have whenever she eats anything containing carbohydrate. Not just sugar (it is a very small relief to learn she doesn't have to avoid sugar, "Although it's best to be sensible," Chrissie tells me. "So if you're going to have sweets, try and have them after meals, when there's something starchy or fatty to slow the effect of the glucose.")

At lunchtime, Chrissie asks Holly what she'd like to eat, and she goes down to the kitchen with her to choose some toast and Marmite, and some crisps, and a chocolate biscuit. We go through a harrowing ten minutes of persuading Holly to have her injection. I have to be firm with her, though I feel like I need to scream and cry, too. In the end, hunger wins, and she allows Chrissie to do what she needs to do.

While Holly eats, Chrissie explains how she worked out the carb content and the amount of insulin required based on a ratio which, she says, will definitely change over time. "But don't worry about that now. You will have so much support and you'll soon figure it out. Honestly, you'll surprise yourself."

It is so much to take in. So much. And all on top of this brand-new knowledge that my daughter has a condition – not an illness, I have already sworn I won't be calling it that, much less a disease – which will be with her forever, and affect every day of her life. My head is an absolute mess. And I still have not been able to speak to Sam. By the time I see his name on my phone screen, I'm worn out.

"What's up?" he asks cheerfully, and I remember he doesn't know anything about all this. I have already taken strides into this new world of which he is completely unaware. I'm about to bring him in.

I take a deep breath.

"We're in hospital," I say flatly.

"What? Why? You and Holly?"

"Yes," I say, and those tears are back, but this time there is no stopping them. I turn away from Holly, who is glued to the TV anyway, seeming none the worse for her recent screaming fit at the injection she was subjected to. "She's got diabetes," I say quietly, although Holly is already fully aware of that fact.

"What? How?"

"I don't know how. Nobody does. It's a weird thing, an autoimmune disease. It's type one, not type two," I say, feeling like I am already becoming an expert, although I suspect in reality I have barely scratched the surface of all there is to know.

"So why are you in hospital? Is she really bad?" I take a moment to answer, aware that I now need to educate Sam a bit about this. Holly could have been very ill, if this hadn't been picked up on when it was. But if Sam means is her diabetes really bad then it is something else which we are going to have to get our heads around. Diabetes just is – there is no 'really bad', but it could be badly managed. I have Chrissie to thank for all of this knowledge. She has sat patiently with me and Holly all afternoon, and explained and re-explained so many things. We are due a visit from a specialist diabetes nurse soon too, and a dietitian.

"Where's Ben?" Sam asks, suddenly worried.

"Your mum's got him," I say. I hadn't really wanted to tell Karen what was going on before I'd told Sam, and before I'd told Mum and Dad – who I couldn't get hold of. But I couldn't very well not tell her, and in fact she was brilliant.

"Oh Alice," she said, "I am so sorry. I know you'll be in shock at the moment. I think I am, too. But listen, my friend Ruthy from school, she's been diabetic since she was fifteen. Type one, too. And she's still very much going strong. Remember that, OK?"

"I will," I had sniffled, grateful for her kind words and feeling guilty that I hadn't expected her to be so immediately supportive and understanding. Chrissie said sometimes people will ask if it's down to a child's lifestyle or diet, or they'll tell you it can be reversed, and she says it drives people mad. I'd been prepared for Karen to be one of these people, but I was wrong.

"Ben will be just fine, we'll have a great time. And maybe when Sam's back he can bring him to see you and Holly; what do you think? He might be worried, it would be good for him to see you. Good for you, too."

"Yes," I said, not really having considered this. But she was right. "Yes, that's a good idea. Thank you so much, Karen."

"It's really no bother, darling," she said, and the 'darling' touched me. She is not normally one for terms of endearment. I had put the phone down and tried again to call Sam but again got no answer. Only now, nearly an hour after I spoke to Karen, have I been able to speak to him. And I realise all of a sudden that he must be in shock, as Karen had said she was, and that the best thing possible would be for us all to be together.

"Can you come here?" I ask, feeling pathetic and small.

"Yes of course," he says. "I'm on my way. Shall I bring Ben?"

"Yes! Bring him. This is going to affect all of us. And Sam?"

"Yes?"

"Take your time. Be safe."

"Of course I will. Love you, Alice."

"I love you too."

Sam sends a message to say he's trying to find somewhere to park, and just as I'm reading it, there's a knock on the door. A friendly-faced woman pokes her head into the room. "Holly and Alice?"

"Yes," I say, with a false cheer in my voice. "That's us."

"I'm Rachel," she says. "The paediatric diabetes specialist nurse. You can just call me Rachel, though. And if you have to use my job title, I'd go with PDSN. It's less of a mouthful."

I smile at her gratefully.

"Mind if I come all the way in?" she asks, smiling at Holly.

"Of course! Please do," I say.

She enters, with a large bag in her hand. "Now you're probably feeling a bit shaken and a bit scared," she says to me. "And Holly, I hear you've had your first injection. That's fantastic!"

I can think of other words to describe it, but I appreciate what she's doing, and I know beyond doubt that we have to try and make this as positive for Holly as we possibly can.

"It hurt," says Holly.

"Ah, I know, it's a bit strange at first, but did you see how small that needle is, on the injection pen?"

Holly shakes her head.

"No? Well, I'll show you. I've got lots of things here to show you, in fact, so that you get to know about diabetes.

There are lots of children who have it, you know, and they tell me that it doesn't take long for it to feel normal. Just part of life. Like brushing your teeth."

Normal? I can't imagine any of this ever feeling normal, but I suppose that it must, at some point. People do live with it, after all. But right now, the thought of it just makes me feel sick. I don't want to learn to live with it. I don't want it to be normal. I want to go back to yesterday, when normal was something else.

She is good, though, Rachel, and she turns to me with a look which shows she knows what I'm thinking, and understands how I'm feeling. "It's true," she says. "I know it probably doesn't even seem real just yet. But look, I've worked with children with diabetes for twelve years now. I've seen lots of new diagnoses. I've seen children grow up and become adults. They take it in their stride, most of these kids. And their parents have to learn to do the same. I think maybe it's harder for the parents sometimes."

I nod, and gulp, feeling those ever-present tears pushing against my eyes.

"Look, Holly, shall we get some of these things out? I've even got a special new friend for you, to have a look at." She pulls a cuddly lion toy out of her bag. "This is Fred, and he's got diabetes too. And he says he doesn't mind if you and Mummy want to practise injections on him. And finger pricks, too. Just till you know how to do them to yourself. Would you like to hold him?"

Holly beams and takes Fred from Rachel. She even remembers to say thank you. I'm grateful to Rachel for taking control of the situation, and giving me a chance to catch my breath. Just as she and Holly are looking at the little device for doing finger-pricks, there is another knock on the door and I say, "Come in."

Sam and Ben step in, both looking a bit nervous.

"I've got a new lion, Daddy!" Holly says, brandishing Fred. "Look!"

"Oh wow, Holly, he's a handsome chap," Sam says, brushing a kiss across the top of my head. "OK?" he murmurs.

"Yes," I say, convincing nobody. "This is Rachel, who's a...?"

"PDSN," she reminds me. "Paediatric Diabetes Specialist Nurse. But you can just call me Rachel. You might be seeing quite a bit of me over the next few weeks."

Sam shakes her hand, and Ben comes across to cuddle me, sliding his way onto my knee.

"Alright?" I ask him.

"What's wrong with Holly?" he asks.

"It's not... there's nothing wrong..." I say, trying to find the right words.

"Your little sister has got something called diabetes," Rachel steps in. "Have you heard of that?"

Ben shakes his head.

"It's Ben, isn't it?" she asks him. He nods. "Well, Ben, diabetes is a.... it's something that happens when a part of a person's body called the pancreas stops working properly. The pancreas produces something called insulin, which helps the body move blood glucose to the parts of the body that need it. Without insulin, the glucose stays in the blood and that can make somebody feel poorly."

"But why?"

"Well, that's a good question. We don't know why people get type one diabetes, which is what Holly has. But we do know that we can use a different type of insulin, to help the body behave the way it's meant to. It just means having to remember to do it, when Holly needs it."

"How do you do that?"

"Another great question! Do you want to tell Ben, Holly?"

"I have injections," Holly says, "like Fred."

"Injections?" Ben looks horrified.

"Yes, but it's not so bad," Rachel clarifies. "Look, we can do an injection on Fred here and you can see how it works. Would you like that?"

Ben nods.

"Great. Then maybe I can show all four of you, and Holly, maybe we can do another finger prick to find out if that injection earlier is helping you. Would that be alright?"

Holly looks uncertain about this.

"It'll be OK, Holly," I say.

"If we do it, then you and Ben could go and play in the playroom for a while. Have you seen the playroom?" Rachel asks.

Holly shakes her head.

"Oh, it's fantastic. And there's a lovely lady called Lisa in there today, she'll show you around. And then I can have a chat with Mummy and Daddy. How does that sound?"

I can see Ben is excited at this idea. Holly is a little more reticent.

"You can do it, Holly," Sam says. "And that playroom sounds amazing!"

While Holly is coming round to the idea, Rachel shows us all the injection pen, and the insulin cartridge and needles – which really are small, I am glad to see, though I still wouldn't want to have to inject myself numerous times a day. Having said that, I'd rather it was me than Holly. She shows us how to do something called an 'air shot' first to make sure there are no bubbles, then how to set the required amount of insulin. I don't know how I'm ever going to remember all of this. What if I do it wrong – or give Holly too much insulin, or not enough? My stomach is churning and I am close to tears yet again.

Thankfully, Holly accepts the prospect of the finger-prick test very gracefully, and Rachel is pleased to see that the number has come down to 9.4.

"Is that still too high?" I ask.

"A little. But it's going the right way. And it takes a bit of time for us to work out the right amount for each person. Everybody's different. We tend to err on the side of caution. Fantastic, Holly – and Ben, too. I'm going to give you both a sticker, then we'll ask Chrissie to take you along to the playroom so that I can have a chat with your mum and dad, OK?"

Both nod, and accept their stickers proudly. In a different setting, amongst his friends, Ben might try to pretend he's not bothered, but here he is free to be a little boy, and I can see he's pleased.

Rachel goes to the door. "Ah, there she is," she says. "Chrissie! These two fantastic children need to go and see the playroom."

Chrissie appears in an instant and smiles at us all,

introducing herself to Sam. "Come on, then," she says to Ben and Holly, "let's go and have some fun, shall we?"

They flank her and I hear Ben chatting to her as they vanish into the ward. And then Sam looks at me, and I put my arms around him. Rachel tactfully gives us a moment, popping out into the ward for a bit.

"What the fuck?" says Sam, into my ear.

"I know," I say miserably. "I can't believe it."

"I thought she'd get some medicine from the doctor and be right as rain by the weekend."

"Me too."

We hold each other, and then Rachel returns, and the hard work begins again. She is so good at explaining everything, and reassures us more than once that this isn't down to anything we've done, or haven't done. It's just plain old bad luck, or genetics, or something. "Nobody really knows yet, exactly what it is that causes it, which makes it incredibly hard to find a cure. But there are plenty of people working on it, all around the world, believe me."

"So it might not be forever?" I ask, hopefully.

"No, it might not. Things change all the time and technology is coming on in leaps and bounds, too. We'll come to that, eventually, but we'll stick with the good old-fashioned finger pricks and injections for the time being, until you've got your heads round it. And while it may not be forever, I'm afraid that at the moment we have to work on the basis that it will be."

Forever. What a word. It's a lovely thing, when it comes to love. Marriage. Friendship. Not when it comes to my four-year-old having diabetes. I stifle a sob.

"Come on," Sam puts his arm around me. "We'll work this out. We can do it. I know we can."

Rachel smiles at him.

"I know," I say, "I'm just gutted. I think my heart's broken."

"It'll mend," he says. "It's not broken, just cracked. And we can fix it."

I am beyond grateful for him and his positivity right now. I can't say I am a hundred per cent convinced, but I hope he is right. And in fact, I think, pulling my shoulders back and pushing my chin up, he has to be. We have to do this. Live with it. Work it out. There is no alternative.

"OK," I say to Rachel. "Let's do this."

There is so much to take in, and so many questions to ask.

"You'll have plenty more," Rachel assures me, "but that is absolutely fine. There are four of us PDSNs and we're on hand all office hours to answer questions. If there's anything that can't wait, you can call the ward here. And I'd suggest you prepare to stay for a few days, till you're confident with everything."

A few days? I suppose it will have to be. Amethi flits into my head. And Julie! I must call her. I need to tell her about this. But she's leaving me, I think, childishly. None of this will affect her, in Canada. I know that's unfair, and not true. She'll be devastated to hear about Holly. But I feel angry at everything and everyone, and the world in general. This is not how life was meant to go.

When we have a fifteen-minute break, I call her. "Alice!" she says. "I'm so happy to hear from you. Lizzie said you're in hospital. With Holly. Is she OK?"

"No," I say. "She's not. She's got diabetes."

There is a moment's pause at the other end of the line. "She's what?"

"She's got diabetes," I say. I am going to have to get used to telling people that.

"Shit."

"Yep."

"What does… what does it mean for her?"

"Oh, she can still live a normal life," I say airily, not wanting to give in to the utter despair that is only inches away. "But she'll have to have injections, every day."

"How many?"

"Five, at least."

"Shit!" she says again.

"I know."

"And I can't believe I've just gone and dropped all that on you about us going away."

"It's fine," I say. "You could hardly not tell me, could you?"

"No," she says, "I know, but it feels like incredibly bad timing, to say the least."

"Yeah, well, shit happens."

"Don't say that."

"I don't mean it quite as it sounded. I just mean that this is life, isn't it? We don't know what's going to occur from one day to the next."

"When are you coming home?" she asks.

"I don't know. It might be a few days."

"Is she really ill?" Julie sounds horrified.

"No, she's not, there's just a lot to learn. To be honest, I

106

don't want to be here, but I'm glad we've got people around who know what they're doing, because I haven't got a clue."

"Well look, first off, don't worry about anything here. We've got everything covered, alright?"

"Thank you," I say, meaning it. I could do without having to consider work right now.

"And we'll talk again, about the Canada stuff. All of that. It's not definite," she offers.

"Don't worry, Julie. You've got to do what's right for your family," I say, having no energy to object to anything. "Honestly."

"Oh Alice." I hear tears in her voice.

"I'll call you later," I say, not able to deal with anybody else's emotions. Besides, I need to tell Mum and Dad.

"Diabetes?" Dad asks. "But Holly's not overweight."

"No, Dad," I say, already realising I may have to go through this numerous times, "it's not that type of diabetes. It's an autoimmune condition. It's just how it is for some people."

"I'll put your Mum on," he manages to mutter, and I can tell he's in tears, too. I feel bad, knowing he is not well. This will hit him hard.

"Alice?" I hear, and I am so glad to hear my mum's voice.

"Mum!" I say, and my tears come freely once more.

"Are you OK? Is Holly?"

"We're fine. Well, kind of. We will be, anyway."

"Did I hear your dad say diabetes?"

"Yes."

"Oh, Alice."

"I know. And we're stuck in hospital for the time being."

107

"Can we bring you anything?"

"I think Sam's got everything for tonight."

"Could we come and see you anyway?"

"Yes, of course. The nurse is here at the moment, going through everything with us. I think visiting hours are a bit later. I can find out."

"Don't worry about that. I'll find out, and your dad and I will come across. I'll let you know when we're on our way. And if it's not convenient, just say."

Despite everything, I feel better for speaking to her. "Thank you, Mum."

By the time Mum and Dad arrive, Holly has had her second meal with an insulin injection. She was very brave, and I decided I should be, too. With Rachel supervising, I did the air shot, and worked out the correct amount of insulin for the number of carbs. And I convinced Holly to let me give her an injection, while she held onto Sam's fingers. "Squeeze as hard as you like, Holly," he said, then, "not that hard... ow!" Making her giggle.

Holly actually watched the needle go into the soft fold of flesh on her belly, and Ben helped to count to ten as instructed by Rachel, then I withdrew the insulin pen, seeing a tiny dot of blood on my daughter's perfect skin. It turned my stomach, but I held my nerve.

"Brilliant, Holly. You are brilliant!" I exclaimed. "And Ben, you were so helpful, thank you."

Both children were beaming, and Rachel was smiling at me too. *This is it, then*, I thought. *This is the way it's going to be from here on in.*

Holly gobbled up her fish fingers, chips and beans. "This often happens, once a child's started on their insulin therapy. Their appetite increases for a while. In fact, there's a honeymoon period, when the body's still probably producing some insulin, and it's a good time to get her eating as much good stuff as possible."

"I'll bear that in mind," I say, adding it to my already ever-growing mental portfolio of diabetes knowledge.

Ben was also allowed to eat with Holly, just this once, and Dad laughs to see the bean sauce on his chin. "Been eating, Benny?" he asks. He looks even more pale and drawn than he has lately.

"How did you know?" Ben exclaims.

"Just a feeling."

Rachel introduces herself; she has stayed to meet Mum and Dad. "If you want to come back tomorrow, I can do some education with you if you'd like to," she offers.

"That sounds great, doesn't it, Phil?" Mum says.

"Yes… yes please." Dad is looking at Holly.

"Go and give her a hug!" I say, and he does. And Mum pulls a couple of parcels from her bag.

"What's that, Granny?" Ben asks, immediately alert.

"We brought you and Holly a little treat," she says, handing Ben a package.

"Jurassic World Lego! Brilliant!" he exclaims. For Holly, there is a Lego Friends set.

We say thanks and bye to Rachel, and Sam fetches us all a drink from the machine nearby, then we take the children down to the playroom, which has a great outside area. The two of them run around, trying out the different scooters and bikes, while we sit quietly, sipping our drinks and talking about the day. Mum and Dad have lots of questions, which I do my best to answer, but to be honest I feel like my brain is saturated, and I'm exhausted from taking it all on board. I need to let it process, I think.

When visiting hours are up, Holly and I have hugs and kisses from Sam, Ben, Mum and Dad, and then they go, and the ward begins to quieten down. Somewhere, there is a baby crying. The sound brings tears to my own eyes – then again, it wouldn't take much at the moment.

I help Holly get changed for bed, and brush her teeth, and then Chrissie comes in before her shift ends, to talk about overnight care, and how we will get into a routine with basal injections, but they want to just monitor Holly's blood glucose overnight. She does another finger-prick test and I'm proud to see Holly already accepting of these. In the space of just a few hours, my little girl has already begun to adapt. I feel like it might take me longer.

In time, Holly drifts off to sleep, and I settle down on my low-level bed next to hers. I am shattered but I know it's going to be difficult to make sleep come. I scroll through Facebook, and Instagram, but I'm irritated by everything, and so I message Sam and tell him I miss him and Ben. His reply is immediate.

We miss you too xx

Are you OK? Xxx

I think so. You? Xxx

I think so. I'll have to be. We all will. Going to try and get some sleep now. I love you xxx

I love you too xxx

I am grateful for him, and for Mum and Dad, and Karen. We have a good solid support structure around us, and I think we're going to need it.

I close my eyes and practise deep, slow breathing, then counting down from 1000 – and get well into the six-hundreds before I fall asleep. Yet somehow, I do.

I am woken by an unfamiliar nurse sometime in the small hours, saying that Holly is having a hypo, which means her blood sugars are too low, and we need to get her to eat something. The nurse wakes her gently and persuades her to eat two jelly babies and then hands me a digestive. "If she eats this it should keep her steady for the rest of the night," she says.

Holly is confused but obedient, tucking into the biscuit without question. The sight and sound of her, half-asleep and munching away in the dim light, makes me so sad, and again I am struck by that word: Forever. This is not something that we can make right with a few nights in hospital. This is forever.

Still, she falls back to sleep, and I step out into the ward, seeing the nurse. She smiles. "Did she eat it?"

"Yes."

"Good girl. I'll come and check on her again in fifteen minutes. Do you need anything? Some water? A hot drink?"

"I wouldn't mind a hot chocolate," I say, thinking maybe it will help me get back to sleep.

"No problem. I'll bring one in a few minutes."

"Thank you so much," I say, tearfully.

"It's no problem." She places a hand on my arm. "It will be OK, you know."

"I know," I say, though I'm not convinced.

"My partner's diabetic."

"Really?"

"Yes, and he's nearly thirty now. He was a similar age to Holly when he was diagnosed. And he's a doctor," she adds with a note of pride in her voice. Despite everything, that makes me smile.

"Thank you," I say. "That's good to hear."

"Go and get back into bed," she says. "I'll be through asap."

I feel the warmth of the hot chocolate running comfortingly through me, and I'm happy that the nurse – Amy, her name tag says – is satisfied that Holly's blood sugar level is back up. Holly sleeps through the whole thing, even the finger-prick.

"Amazing!" I smile.

"Kids do this," she says. "Parents say they can give their children jelly babies to treat night-time hypos and in the morning the kids don't remember a thing!"

"Bloody hell," I say, contemplating having to deal with this kind of thing at home.

"I know! But," she says, no doubt seeing the worry on my face, "if Holly goes onto an insulin pump at some point, it will make night times a lot easier. It's so much right now, I know it is. You'll get there. I promise."

An insulin pump? At the moment I can't even begin to get my head around what that is. I think Amy realises this. "Try and get some sleep," she says kindly.

When she's gone, I finish my hot chocolate and go into the bathroom to clean my teeth again. I look in the mirror and see a pale, drawn face looking back at me. There are dark circles under my eyes. I need to sleep. I will need all the energy I can get.

Tiptoeing back into the room, I stop next to Holly, and listen to her breathing. I kiss her forehead and place my finger into her hand so that she grips it for a while. Then I ease it slowly out and get back into the squeaky-clean bed, hoping that sleep will come easily and I can slide into oblivion for a few merciful hours.

12

In the end, Holly and I spend three long, restless nights in hospital. It feels like much longer, but I am very grateful for it all. Having the safety net of nurses coming in and checking on Holly, and people to ask for support, is worth any amount of lost sleep. By the time we're ready to leave, I'm feeling attached to Chrissie, and Amy, and Rachel – three people who this time last week were strangers, but who have just been with me through the most intense experience of my life to date.

"I feel nervous," I tell Chrissie.

"You don't need to be. You're doing great. You and Holly, and Mr Branvall, of course."

Sam and Ben have been in every day. Sam offered to spend one of the nights here, but I couldn't bring myself to leave Holly, even though it would have been her dad with her. I just couldn't do it. And it sounded like he and Ben had been coping OK.

"Zinnia came round for tea yesterday," Ben said, on the second morning we were here.

"Did she?" My mind flitted to Julie, who had been in regular contact via WhatsApp, but who I had been providing with only minimal responses. Horrible though it sounds, I can't seem to shake this resentment towards her.

There she is, planning a new future with her husband, and her perfectly healthy little girl. They have no money worries to speak of, either. Julie once told me she wouldn't have to work if she didn't want to – though she assured me that she did want to. And that she loved Amethi every bit as much as I do. I can't help but doubt the truth of that now.

And yet… I know she's had hard times. She was fatherless growing up. Her mum, Cherry, struggled sometimes, to keep Julie and her brother Lee fed and clothed, and at the same time ensure that they had a warm, safe house in which to sleep. Then there were Julie and Luke's struggles to conceive. I know that I'm being mean and unfair but right now it's how I feel.

David has also been in regular contact and he and I have spoken a couple of times. He also immediately volunteered to help at Amethi if needed, but Lizzie seems to have that side of things covered.

"Are you sure?" David had asked. "I quite like the idea of hospitality. I think it might suit me."

"I could see that," I said, "and if I was there to show you the ropes, it would be brilliant. But, call me a control freak, I would want to know that anybody gets the way things are done at Amethi before letting them loose on the place."

"Control freak," he said, and I could tell he was grinning. "And anyway, what do you mean, 'let me loose'? I'm not a dog."

Each call with David has cheered me up a bit. And he's also somebody who has a friend with diabetes – and a colleague, too. It's good to hear stories of adults who have come safely through childhood with diabetes, and are now living successful, happy lives.

What is also immensely cheering is that David no longer has to worry about that parent from school. Apparently, the man realised that there would be nothing to gain financially, and he's been in trouble with the law himself on one or two occasions, and didn't want to get too close to it all again.

"Basically, he couldn't be arsed!" David laughs, but I can tell he's relieved.

"So you didn't need to leave your job, though?"

"Well, no, but things have a habit of working themselves out."

When Holly and Ben were in the play area, I ask Sam about Zinnia coming for tea. "Yes, they all came," he said, and he looked at me meaningfully. "Why didn't you say anything?"

"They told you, then?"

"Yes. Julie said you were upset."

"Of course I'm upset!" I responded angrily. "She's leaving me." I felt myself opening up like the sky in a thunderstorm, and I leaned into Sam, who just put his arms around me and let me cry.

"Your shirt's wet," I said after a while, dabbing at the place that my tears had dampened.

"Oh, that's just great," he said, but he was smiling.

"Sorry," I sniffled.

"Oh Alice," he said, and I could see his eyes were gleaming.

"Don't you feel like that, about Luke?" I asked.

"Not really. I mean, I'll miss him, of course. He's my best mate. After you, of course. But I think it's a good idea."

"Do you?"

"Yes, or at least I can see why they want to do it. It's too painful for Luke, being here, without his parents. And you know what he's like. He's got a sense of adventure. So's Julie. You always say that about her."

"Not like us boring pair," I said, tightening my arms around his middle.

He kissed me on my head. "I don't think we're boring. I think we're just where we want to be."

"But I thought Julie was, too," I half-wailed, feeling pathetic even as the words escaped my mouth.

"And she is, or she was. But it's not just about her, is it? It's Luke, and it's Zinnia. Just like I've got to think of you and Ben and Holly."

"And I've got to think of you three, too," I said. "I know, you're right. But I can't bear to think of life without Julie."

"She'll still be your best mate. And don't worry, you don't have to say after me. I know my place."

That at least made me smile. "Yes, but she'll be thousands of miles away."

"Then we'll have to go and visit."

"It's not the same."

"No, it's not," Sam said firmly, "but it's the best option we've got."

I needed him to say that, really. Because Sam was right. And I was being a silly, snivelling, selfish idiot. But even though I know that, I am still struggling to communicate with Julie. And having Holly's situation at the forefront of my mind is a good excuse not to.

Now it's the third day we have woken up here, and I've been waiting for the OK to leave. I am both excited and nervous about it, but with everything I have learned over the last few days, I feel halfway confident that we can manage back in the outside world, and I am also very keen to prove that this is the case.

With a whole load of kit packed safely away, and forms signed – not to mention a raft of appointments made for the coming weeks – Holly and I are ready. As I'd brought my car along when we came here – which seems like weeks, not days, ago – I've told Sam not to worry about coming in, and that Holly and I will be home as soon as we can be.

It's strange, driving back, making the journey in reverse. I wish I could reverse all the way back through the days, but I have to stop thinking like that. I need to reprogramme my mind, because there is nothing I can do to change the fact Holly has diabetes. The only thing I can control is the way that I cope with it, and the way that I communicate with Holly and Ben about it. This cannot be a terrible thing for them. It has to just be. Rachel's told me about a family support group, and suggested we might want to go to one of their events, but I don't know. I just want us to slot back into life as normally as possible.

Holly sleeps all the way. She is wiped out by our time in hospital; we both are. I catch glimpses of her via the central mirror, and see her sweet little head lolling against the side of her car seat. *This is it, Alice,* I tell myself. *This is your chance to make this normal for Holly, and for Ben. It's not about you.*

I think that is a key thing. It is not about me. It is going to affect me, every day – I can already see that – but it's my responsibility as a parent to make this alright for my children. As much as it's my responsibility to make sure Holly has her insulin when she needs it, I need to make sure she also has the right attitude towards it all.

When I draw up at our house, I am ready to just carry Holly in and flop down on the settee, but I see we have visitors. Julie, Luke and Zinnia.

"Hello," I say stiffly, as I enter the hallway to see my friend there instead of Sam. I don't know how to feel about her being there.

"Alice," she says, stepping forward to envelop me and Holly in a hug. I accept it stiffly, but I don't return it − for one thing, my arms are around Holly, who is still sleepy. She, however, turns and puts her arms around Julie. My friend looks to me for permission, and I shrug, so she takes my daughter from me.

"How are you, Miss Holly? Are you glad to be home?"

"Yes," Holly says, but she proceeds to tell Julie about the room she had in hospital, and the play area, and the paintings she's done. She makes it sounds like she's been away on an activity holiday.

Julie carries Holly through to the kitchen and I walk into the lounge. Luke comes in, a cup of tea in his hand. He offers it to me.

"Thank you," I say gratefully, sitting on the settee, which has never felt so comfortable.

Luke sits down on the other side of the seat. He looks at me, concern written over his face. "You must be knackered."

"I am." I thought I'd felt it before, but now I am actually home, it's increased a hundred-fold.

"What can we do to help?" he asks.

I laugh drily. "I don't know. Probably nothing." It is ungracious of me, but there we are.

"Julie's been reading up on it all," he says. "She already knew about the carb-counting thing, and she's done you a load of meals. They're in the freezer, labelled up." I can tell he knows things aren't right between me and her.

"That's really kind," I say, and I mean it.

"And," he says, seizing on the positive note, "we want to help you and Sammy out. We'll have the kids when we can, try and give you a full night's sleep every now and then."

"While you're still here," I say. It's horrible of me.

"Yes. While we're still here." I can see he's not quite sure how to respond. By rights, he should tell me not to be so bloody selfish, but he can see I'm a broken woman right now, and he's too kind and too soft to say that to me anyway. Instead, he changes tack. "You're probably wondering where Ben and Sam are."

"Well, yes, the thought had crossed my mind." I can feel a headache brewing. I just want to go upstairs, pull the curtains closed, and hide under my duvet. I want Holly by my side as well, though. I need to know she's alright.

"They'll be back soon," was all Luke would say. "Sam asked us to be here, in case you got back before they did."

"OK…"

"Anyway, drink your tea. We can keep an eye on Holly."

"I probably need to check her blood sugar," I say pointedly.

"Of course, yes," Luke says, uncertainly. "Can you drink your tea first, though? Just relax a bit?"

"Not really, no. It's not as simple as that." I'm being off with him, completely unreasonably, and actually it could probably wait until I've had my cup of tea. But I want them to see what it's like. What life is going to be like from now on. I stand up and go to my bag, fishing out the clear plastic bags of kit.

"I need to put the insulin in the fridge as well," I say, going into the kitchen.

"Hi Alice!" says Zinnia.

"Hello Zinnie." Despite everything, I can't help but smile at the sight of Luke and Julie's daughter helping mine do some colouring-in. It thaws my unwarranted iciness a touch.

"What's all that?" asks Julie, looking at my bag.

I want to make some comment about it being all the shit that comes with diabetes. But Holly is there, and I need to stick to that promise I made myself. "It's all the kit they sent home from hospital isn't it, Holly? Shall we show Julie and Zinnia how to test your blood sugars?"

"Yes," Holly says, and her enthusiasm is heart-breaking. She proudly shows them how to do a finger-prick blood test, and we all watch the little machine count down. 6.4.

"Is that good?" asks Julie.

"Yes. It's very good. Between 4 and 7 is ideal. But," I say, not wanting her to think it's straightforward, "it can change. It might go low, or it might go high. If it's low, Holly needs some sweets, don't you, darling?"

"And if it's high I need to drink water," Holly says, "and run around, unless I've got ketones."

Julie looks at me. I nod. "That's just the basics," I say.

"I want to know. I want to learn," Julie tells me, earnestly.

"I want to help you guys."

Unlike with Luke, I don't make any disparaging comments. I just look at my friend's face and remember why she means so much to me. "Thank you," I say. "That would be great."

I do then sit and drink my tea, and then I hear a key in the door. Meg runs through first, greeting Holly and me excitedly. Then I hear Ben's voice. "They're back, Daddy!"

He runs through and I sweep him up into a huge hug. "I've missed you! Have you been growing?"

"Don't know!" he giggles.

Then Sam comes in. He hugs first Holly, and then me. "Sorry we weren't here when you got back."

"That's OK. But where were you?"

"We've been on a mission haven't we, Ben?"

"Yes! To make our house better."

"I didn't know it was poorly."

"No, silly. Better for Holly, and for you."

I look at Sam. "I was thinking about the things that might be difficult, and what we might be able to do about them. For one thing, we've been saying for ages we need a bigger fridge-freezer. And when Julie started delivering all these amazing meals – you have told her about them, haven't you?" He looks to Julie for confirmation. She nods. "Well, when this amazing friend of yours started turning up with millions of takeaway boxes, I realised we didn't have space for them. So Ben and I have ordered a new fridge freezer, twice as big as this one. Haven't we, Benny?"

"Yes, and we got Holly a new bed, too."

"Did you?"

"Yes, a big one, like mine, so if you or Daddy need to stay in with her there's room for you to lie down too."

My eyes fill with tears.

"You don't mind, do you?" asks Sam. "That we haven't waited for you?"

"No," I say, "of course I don't mind. I'm just… incredibly grateful. To all of you." I hug them each in turn, and I ask Julie to show me the meals she's brought.

I am blown away − Sam may have been exaggerating slightly, but there are enough to keep us going for days. And each one is labelled with what's in it, what a portion size is, and how much carbohydrate is in a portion. It doesn't take much to set me off at the moment, and predictably the sight of all this has me in tears. "Bloody hell, Julie," I sniffle. "This is incredible."

"It's not − not really. It's what I do, isn't it? Food, I mean."

"Yes, but it must have taken you ages."

"I just wanted to help, and it seemed to me that this might be the best way to do it. You've got enough to contend with right now, at least you won't have to think about cooking, too. Let's face it, we know it's not your strong suit."

I let out a surprised laugh, which I realise might be my first real laugh in days. It feels good.

"Rub it in, why don't you?" I link my arm through hers, and I can see both Sam and Luke look relieved at the sight.

"Your mum and dad were going to come, Alice, but I put them off till tomorrow. Is that OK?" Sam asks.

"Yes, I think so. I think we just need to get back into being at home. And get used to things at our own pace."

"Which is our cue to leave," says Julie.

"I didn't mean it like that. You're welcome to stay…"

"No, no, I know you didn't. But you're right. You four, and Meg, need some time together now." She has a job of persuading Zinnia, who wants to stay, and Ben doesn't help, by adding his voice in protest, but soon my friend and her family are at the front door.

"Thank you, all of you," I say. "Honestly."

"It's nothing, Alice. And you just tell us when you need us, OK? I want to know how it all works, and what to do, so you and Sam don't feel on your own with this."

When they've gone, I stand in the quiet hallway for a moment, and I hear Meg's nails clicking gently on the hard floor, then I feel her push her nose into my hand. I hear Sam and the kids chatting in the kitchen, so I crouch and stroke my dog, pressing my face into her fur, and allowing myself a few quiet, unseen tears, before I return to the kitchen and the reality of this new way of living.

13

At first, it seemed like nothing would ever seem normal again. And as summer began to present itself – ironically, the weather improved almost as soon as we were back from the hospital, and town began to fill up with holiday-makers and day-trippers – I felt sad that I wouldn't be able to enjoy it as I normally do. I felt like I might never quite be able to enjoy anything properly again.

I hated it, the finger pricks, the injections, Holly's tears. I dreaded that first hypo at home, when Holly's blood sugars fell, but after a couple of jelly babies she was soon right as rain again. And I couldn't rest at night, needing to know that she was OK.

"You can't keep on checking on her," Sam said. "Not as much as you are doing. She won't sleep properly, and you won't rest at all."

"She sleeps through it all," I said, annoyed, feeling like he was criticising me.

"That's as may be, but listen to what Rachel's telling you. We know where we are with it all a bit more now. And even though Holly seems to sleep through, it might still be disturbing her."

I knew he was right, of course, but it seemed impossible to rest unless I knew what her blood sugars were. At first, we were asked to check on her every two hours, to make sure she was steady overnight, and we knew that we had her basal doses more or less right, but once we seemed to have achieved success, Rachel said we could reduce this to every four hours, and then to eight. Meaning we should all have been able to get some sleep. But that was easier than it sounds. Because what if she became ill overnight?

I would lie awake, worrying about her, and eventually creep in to see her. It was like an addiction, and I had to actively fight the urge to do a finger-prick test on her. Once I'd managed to conquer that, and felt a little bit more confident that we would all wake up in the morning, my fears changed to what ifs. What if we hadn't got Holly to the doctors when we did? She could have been seriously ill, or worse. What if we didn't have access to the NHS and their incredible support, not to mention free supply of insulin and blood test strips and all the other equipment we have been so fortunate to receive? What if we lived in a place like war-torn Syria, the Yemen, or Ukraine? How do people in places like that lay their hands on these things? I would imagine having to leave our home, and how impossible that would be.

Over the weeks, these thoughts have died down a little, but the fear is never far from the surface. It feels like it is just a matter of putting one foot wrong, and it could spell disaster. But this is a way of thinking that I need to overcome. I am starting to tell myself that living with a condition like diabetes isn't so different to living without it. There are things that everyone needs to do, and not do, to live. When you have diabetes – and I guess many other conditions –

there are just more of these things, and some are more immediately crucial. It just means being on the case at all times.

And now, as we are approaching the summer solstice, and Ben's birthday, I feel slightly more on top of it all. A little more confident that we can do this. I no longer feel that some kind of disaster is necessarily imminent.

Also, I have Sam to share the responsibility – and support from Julie, Luke, Mum, Dad and Karen – although Dad is struggling still himself, and I can see on his face when he looks at Holly that he is distressed about her having to live with diabetes. I understand it, I feel it too – we all do – but it's not helpful to let on to Holly, or Ben, how anxious we are.

"I wish you'd let us help more, Alice," Mum has said, more than once.

"I know, Mum," I've told her, "and we will. You will. You already are, in fact–" Mum has learned about carb-counting, and she's bought a diabetes cookbook, from which she regularly brings us cakes and cookies to try (some are better than others) – "but you and Dad still need to sort your own stuff out."

With the Sail Loft on the market, it could be only a matter of time before they have to finalise their move, and so we are all keeping an eye out for bungalows for them. It gives me something else to think about – as does work, because now Holly's nursery carers have been trained by Rachel, they are also able to do her injections, etc. and I can let Holly enjoy her last few weeks there before she leaves to start at school. It was quite a wrench, handing over the responsibility to somebody else, but it's probably no bad thing. Being at work is good for my mental health – if I concentrate on the here and now, and don't look too far ahead – and knowing that I am not the only person who can do what Holly needs is important.

It's so strange how everything has changed, and yet nothing has. My whole world seems completely different to me, and I feel like I want that acknowledged in some way but actually, everything carries on much as before. Nursery for Holly, school for Ben, work for me and Sam. It's good, really – I do realise that – and in fact incredibly important, that life is normal for all of us. I don't want Holly feeling like having diabetes is going to be a reason to change the way we live, or which should stop her doing anything she wants to do, but I feel personally fundamentally changed in some way. I wanted to cancel my evening with Lydia, but Sam had insisted I go, and I'm glad that he did.

We went out for an Italian, and it was just so good to sit and chat and eat, and drink a couple of glasses of red wine.

It was also good to listen to Lydia, as she needed somebody to speak to, and although I wouldn't wish any of the problems she's experiencing on her, it was kind of a nice change to have somebody else's issues to focus on.

"It's that bloody agent. *Xavier*," she said exasperatedly, taking a gulp of wine and glaring into the glass as if she might find the root of her problems there. "But it's Si as well. *Xav* is pushing him around, and trying to control him – Si's just letting him. He should be sticking up for himself. Do you know, he doesn't even want to do that bloody film in

America? He never wanted to work over there – but Xav says it's vital for his career."

"Surely that's up to Si?" I asked, aware that I know absolutely nothing about the film and TV industry, but nevertheless imagining that it would be hard to pass up on an opportunity to 'break America', as they say.

"Well, yes, you'd think, wouldn't you? Vital for his career–" she repeated, bitterly – "more like vital for Xavier's career. And bank balance."

"I wish I could help," I said.

"You are doing, just listening, thank you, Alice. And I'm sorry, I know life's really hard for you at the moment."

"It's fine," I said, "honestly. It's nice not to be thinking about Holly, or Dad, for a while."

"They're really selling the Sail Loft?" she asked.

"Yes. Sad, isn't it? But also the right thing for them to do. You don't fancy buying it, do you?" I asked, smiling.

"Ha! I wouldn't mind. I don't think it's very realistic."

"Well if Si's doing this film, he should be able to buy it for you!"

"Don't even joke about it," she said grimly. "Honestly, if he does go, and it looks like he will, then I don't know if we've really got a future."

"You definitely wouldn't go with him?"

"No. I just… it's not me. And I'm at home here. I like it. Love it, in fact. I want to be here. My family's here. My work's here. My friends are here. I feel so uncomfortable in Si's world."

"But not with Si," I say.

"No, not when it's just me and him."

129

The waiter brought us the dessert menus. "Shall we?" Lydia raised her eyebrows at me.

"Why not?"

"This is my treat, by the way," she said. "I'm just so grateful to have somebody I can talk to who I can trust."

"And you can. Trust me, and talk to me. Any time."

I used to feel quite maternal towards Lydia, when she was a young part-time waitress at the Sail Loft – even though there is really only a handful of years between us. Now I suppose she feels more like a younger sister. I certainly feel protective of her, and I don't like the sound of this agent of Si's.

We chatted more over dessert, and she asked me lots of questions about diabetes, which I appreciated, but I'd been keen to keep the focus on her. I didn't even tell her about Julie's plans. I still wasn't sure what to say or think about that.

"So what do you think you're you going to do?" I asked, clarifying, "About Si."

"Well, it's kind of up to him as well, isn't it? I've told him I want to stay here, and that I do want to be with him. He's coming down in a few weeks, once he's finished the job up in Scotland. I guess that will be a chance for us to talk it through properly. It's much easier talking in person than on the phone, or on a bloody video call."

"Yeah, you should bring him to this place. It's really lovely. And it's tucked away as well. You might be able to get here unnoticed, and actually have a peaceful evening together."

"Isn't it ridiculous, having to think like that? Honestly, I do really like Si – maybe even love him," she admitted, which is quite a thing for Lydia, "but is it enough? I hate having to live looking over my shoulder, and I hate having this outside influence on our lives, with Xavier calling the shots. He's such a patronising prick as well."

"I'm building up quite an image of this bloke."

"It still won't be as bad as the reality," she frowned.

"I just hope you manage to sort it out. You and Si are good together."

"We'll see."

We hugged goodbye outside the restaurant, and Lydia walked back to her flat. I had parked at the Island car park and after checking in with Sam that all was well with Holly, I took the longer route back to the car, down the steep stone steps that pass the tiniest beach in town. The tide was in, and I stopped for a few moments, watching the rippling water illuminated by the lights of the nearby buildings and harbour, and listening to the waves lapping against the base of the old stone walls and the shelf of rocks down below. It was a cloudy night and once the lights could reach no further across the water, there was just thick, inky blackness. Imagining what might lie and move below that velvety surface, I breathed long and slow, hoping for a kind of connection somehow. Something that could create some meaning. I am past the point where I think that everything in life happens for a reason. I used to believe that when I was younger, but now I think that things just happen. But I do believe that if I cast back far enough, I might just find something somewhere, somehow. Some reassurance. A correlation, between the past and the present and the future.

I thought of how Lydia would find it hard to even do what I was doing, stopping to gaze across the bay, without worrying that she'd be snapped. And I thought of Sam at home, and Holly and Ben tucked up in bed.

Those few moments to myself were a luxury, but I needed them. I headed home relaxed, and very full. And when I got back, there was a note from Sam telling me all was well, and noting Holly's blood sugar level. I crept into Ben's room and sat by his bed for a moment or two, kissing his clammy forehead, then I did the same with Holly, trying very hard to stop the twisting in my stomach at the thought of what was happening with her. Finally, I snuck into our bedroom, seeing Sam was already asleep. I got changed in the bathroom and then tiptoed across the soft carpet, sinking gratefully into our bed.

14

"Your last Amethi solstice!" I say to Lizzie, sadly.

"I know. But I'm blessed to have had so many." Typical Lizzie. Always finding the positive. "And we'll make this one extra special. OK?"

"OK." What else can I say? And I surprise myself by realising I am genuinely looking forward to it, and to Ben's birthday. I want to make sure that is extra special too, as he is suddenly having to deal with Holly needing far more attention, and all the painful mealtimes as I try not to watch anxiously to make sure she eats everything. If she's had her insulin and then decides she doesn't want what I've cooked, I have to scrape around to find something else, and I don't want to give in to offering biscuits as a quick fix; it won't take her long to cotton on to that one.

Meanwhile, Julie has not said much more about Canada, but I know it's not going away. And the plans are still very much in place for the surprise anniversary party for her and Luke – so they'd better not be going before then. I'm feeling very twitchy about everything but it's also great to have so many things to think about other than bloody diabetes.

Sam has insisted that I participate in the solstice yoga sessions, and the evening meals, and let him take care of things at home. "It will do you good, Alice. And I'll call if there's any problem, OK? Just work on the notion that no news is good news."

"What have I done to deserve you?" I asked, kissing him.

"I have no idea. Now go on, before I change my mind."

So I am at Amethi with Lizzie to welcome everyone as they arrive, and Julie is busy in the kitchen, cooking up the opening night feast. If I don't think too hard, all feels well with the world. Almost normal.

We have the usual talk from Lizzie, but I have asked not to speak this time, as I genuinely don't know if I have it in me. Luckily, empathic Lizzie had already anticipated this. She merely tells people who Julie and I are, and she says she will be the first port of call for any queries while the retreat is running. I smile at her gratefully, and as the evening gets underway, with a quiet, gentle yoga session, then Julie's five-bean chilli and plenty of rice and tortilla chips, not to mention the gorgeous summery drinks that Lizzie has concocted, I am aware of a fuzzy feeling, as though positivity is seeping into me. The drive back is under a still-light sky, and I see thin stretches of cloud above the horizon. I stop in a layby for a very short time, open my window, and breathe it all in.

By the time I get home, Sam, Holly and Ben are all fast asleep. Meg wakes to greet me, but only briefly. I take a glass of water up to my room, and get changed quietly in the bathroom, brushing my teeth and then sliding under the covers next to Sam. For the first night in a long time, I enjoy a peaceful, heavy, and undisturbed sleep.

***

As I try to focus on Lizzie's soothing voice and her kind, calm words, my mind keeps pulling me in other directions – contemplating how just a few weeks ago I felt like the bottom had fallen out of my world, yet now here I am lying on a yoga mat in the Mowhay, surrounded by some familiar faces; a few of our guests have come back year after year. I don't want to tell them that they won't be able to book next year's retreat as I don't know that there will actually be one.

Breathe, Alice. Be in the moment. Lizzie is not actually transmitting these thoughts to me, or at least I don't think she is. I'm just trying to remind myself of what it is I need to do. It's hard, though; my mind is a jumble of so many anxieties and concerns, and uncertainties. Somebody somewhere snores, and I try not to laugh. I know that next to me, Julie will be the same. I want to open my eyes, turn my head, and grin at her. Ever the silly schoolgirls. It's just one reason I can't bear the thought of her going. Nobody else can ever come close to filling her place in my life.

"Now, start to find a little movement in your hands and feet." I hear Lizzie's actual voice speak into the quiet of the room. Around me, there is gentle shuffling, stretching and turning, and Lizzie continues, "Now open your eyes, slowly, becoming accustomed to the light once more. The sacred light of this most beautiful day. Blink a few times. Let it in. And when you're ready, turn gently onto your left side, before you come back to sitting."

We do as we are told and gradually we are all facing each other in a circle, blinking as we adjust to the real world again.

Lizzie sits in the middle. "It's just a few hours now until our final evening meal, and it's a chance for you all to take some time for yourselves or, if you'd like, you can join me in a barefoot meditation walk along the outskirts of the wildflower fields."

This is new, and I have a feeling it is part of Lizzie's farewell to Amethi. It fills me with sadness, to think of her going, although I am pleased for her, and I know that my sadness is compounded by the thought of another imminent departure. I turn to look at Julie and she smiles at me. She knows what I'm thinking. She's thinking it, too.

We join Lizzie on her walk, as do the majority of our guests. She leads the way slowly, talking softly, and stopping regularly. Meg has accompanied us, seeming to appreciate the slow pace as a chance to stop and smell the hedgerows and animal passages which have flattened the grass in places.

"As we walk, I want you to bring your awareness to each step you take, each muscle you are moving in order to lift your foot and bring it down again. Feel the softness, and the prickles, of the grass that you are stepping on. I do have to say, keep an eye out for stinging insects in particular, but try to focus on your feet. How they feel as they make contact with the ground. You are connecting with the earth in the most simple, joyous, honest way."

Julie takes my hand as we walk, just gently scooping her fingers around mine. I don't look at her, but I focus on the feel of her skin on mine as well; drinking it in, storing it up in my memory bank for those coming days when we won't be together. An image springs to mind of the time we went to collect our GCSE results; her hand in mine back then, too. So many times, over the years; a simple squeeze of each other's fingers, for strength, or sympathy, or to calm nerves – sometimes even to celebrate a success. The power of the human touch. There is no number of Zoom calls that can ever replace this.

When we reach the edge of the woodland, Lizzie asks us all to stop, and listen. Julie and I stand shoulder to shoulder. The sounds are familiar to me, but form a unique combination. There is little breeze today, so the trees stay still and silent, confident and sure of themselves, hosting the little township of birds and insects which flit and crawl between their branches and leaves while small mammals scurry around their feet. I watch a thick-bodied moth fly up from the ground, into the safe cover of leaves in a nearby tree. Just behind Lizzie, a tiny dunnock drops to the ground, hopping around and pecking at the dirt. I close my eyes, to hear more clearly, and the softest breeze whispers across me, just brushing the surface of my skin; my cheeks, and bare shoulders. I feel the ground beneath my feet, rougher now as the grass has given way to bare earth scattered with tree litter. Beside me, Julie's shoulders drop slightly, and I take a long, deep breath, slowly rolling my own shoulders back and down. Letting Amethi work its magic.

We are a happy group heading back, and as the guests split away to their accommodation and Lizzie goes over to get things ready for the evening, I follow Julie into the kitchen.

"That was really special," I say, leaning against one of the counters.

"It was." She has her back to me, pulling some beeswax-wrapped dishes out of the fridge.

"I'm going to miss you."

"I know." She turns. "I am going to miss you, too. And this. We're so lucky, Alice, to have it, and I can't believe I'm giving it up. What am I doing?" she asks suddenly, looking anguished.

"You're doing the best thing for your family," I say.

"Am I, though? We're leaving a place we know and love, with an amazing support network around us. We must be mad."

"I don't know about that. But I think it's one of those things you have to do. If you change your minds now, I think you'll regret it." What am I doing, persuading her to go? This could be my chance to keep her here. But deep down, I know that is not the right thing. Not really.

"Do you really think that?"

"I don't know! It just sounded good." I laugh, and she does, too.

"I just can't bear the thought that this time next year I won't be here."

I don't know what to say. The reality is, I might not be, either. How can I run this place without Julie? She is an integral part of Amethi, and I can't imagine working with anyone else the way I work with her. On a practical level, there is no way that I can afford to keep it by myself. We are scraping by as it is, financially, and time will tell whether people will be willing to pay increased prices to stay here. I don't know. I have some big decisions to make, but I have no idea what they are, or how I go about reaching them. I don't tell Julie that, though; now is not the time. Instead, I put my arms around her, and let her lean her head on my shoulder.

"What will I do without you, Alice?" I hear her muffled words.

"You will have an amazing time," I say firmly. "And you'll never be without me. We will just be in different places, but I'll always be here. Well, not necessarily right here in the kitchen, but I will always be in your life, as long as you want me to be."

My shoulder feels damp, and I realise my strong, independent, sure-minded friend is crying. This is a role-reversal for us. I'm the one given to letting out my emotions, while Julie normally keeps a cool, calm head.

"Sorry," she says. "I blame Lizzie. She's unlocked my weak side."

"Not weak," I say. "Pathetic."

That makes her chuckle, which was my intention. She stands back, and looks at me.

"I want to say the same to you, but I just can't."

"You can."

"Nah. Not right now. Not after the last few weeks. Bloody hell, Alice. Why did nobody ever tell us that being grown up is so hard?"

"I think they probably did – we just didn't listen. Anyway, we need to crack on, my friend. The solstice won't wait for us. Put me to work, please."

And so she does. With Julie giving instructions, I take various dishes and wooden boards through to the dining table in the Mowhay, ready for Julie's mouth-watering food. Outside, Lizzie already has the fire going. She is crouching next to it, gazing at it with such intensity that I dare not disturb her.

Instead, I set about arranging the plates and the flower garlands, making sure that Lizzie's mandala has centre-stage. With sunflowers, roses, camomile and lavender, the air smells beautifully sweet.

Tonight, Julie has kept the food simple, with tomato-and-cheese pastry pinwheels, falafel, samosas, plump and juicy olives, fresh focaccia bread, houmous, tzatziki, and huge bowls of salads. There are jugs of blueberry lavender lemonade, and bottles of elderflower pressé. As our guests come in, exclaiming at everything, we pass the drinks around, and we take it in turns to raise a toast.

Lizzie begins: "This is a special day – the solstice marks the turning of the year and the start of summer proper. But this particular solstice is bittersweet, as it will be the last one I spend here—" the announcement receives a slight gasp of surprise tinged with disappointment – "but I want to celebrate, not commiserate. The welcome these two women gave me when I first turned up here and they probably thought I was some mad old hippy, well I'll never forget it."

I think back to that first vision of Lizzie I had as she stepped out of her car, clad in a full-on poncho, her frizzy hair like a halo around her head. She had come recommended by Kate – Sam's ex, and Sophie's mum. I wondered what she had let us in for, and if I am honest, I had even briefly wondered if she had set us up, secretly still bitter at me. But time showed us Lizzie's true worth and over the years she has become a central figure in my life. She was even instrumental in Holly's birth. I smile, remembering, and Lizzie smiles back at me.

"This has been more than a place of work to me; it's been a home. And not just because of the cottage I've lived so happily in. I've felt like I have belonged here. And I am sure you will agree that to belong in such a special place is a privilege. So I'd like to raise my glass to Julie, and Alice, and Amethi."

Our guests echo the toast and Julie and I both look at each other, embarrassed but pleased.

I take the mantel before I have a chance to well up. "Lizzie," I say, "it has been a pleasure. I can't speak for Julie, but I know that I have learned so much from you. So thank you, Lizzie, for coming here, and for being a part of Amethi... and for being you."

I raise my glass and then sit hurriedly down. Julie takes this as her cue.

"At the risk of this becoming an over-emotional love-in," she says, "I would like to echo Alice's feelings about Lizzie – and Lizzie's feelings about Amethi. This truly is a special place, and we have had so many unforgettable times here. Thanks in part to Lizzie, and in even larger part to Alice, and of course to all of you who put your faith in us to make these times happen."

I had wondered if she was going to mention her plan to leave, but I'm glad that she doesn't. The focus here should still be the solstice, and the event we are running, and this is a chance to celebrate Lizzie's role in it all. Julie has played it exactly right. When we raise our glasses, I raise mine to her. She manages a wobbly smile.

When Lizzie asks if anyone is staying by the fire with her, it is usually my cue to leave. More often than not, she is on her own in this, which she doesn't mind at all. But this year it's different. Julie and I look at each other. We know what to do.

"I'm staying with you, Lizzie," says Julie.

"And I am too!"

Our lovely friend looks shocked and delighted, which tells me immediately that we're doing the right thing. There is a large part of me that is desperate to go home, as I am finding it quite a struggle being away from Holly, and not being there to make sure she's doing OK – although Sam is keeping me updated. I know he will be taking great care of her. It's just very difficult not being there.

It was Sam who suggested that I stay up at Amethi tonight. He knows it's a special one and, he said, "You need to know it's not all down to you. Looking after Holly – and Ben, of course. I can do it too, OK?"

"OK," I had conceded, reluctantly, fighting the control-freak side of myself. And now that I'm here, with the prospect of a night of freedom stretching ahead, I'm just a little bit excited. Of course, the sensible thing would be to grab this opportunity with both hands and get some bloody sleep. But the sensible option is not always the right one. As the guests drift away, as I had hoped they might – I really wanted to spend this time with just my friends, but of course I could not say that out loud – I huddle into the blanket Lizzie has wrapped around my shoulders, and I gaze into the flames.

The night is kind and, despite the clear, star-speckled sky, relatively warm. Coupled with the heat from the fire, I feel toasty, and as relaxed as I have been in some time. I just have to try not to think too hard about… well, anything… and enjoy this little moment in time for what it is.

We talk a little, about the last few days, and how well the retreat has gone. And we reminisce about the first ever time we worked together, and other events we've run across the years. I remember when Lizzie asked us to write down our wishes, and send them to the universe via the flames of the fire. I had written 'happiness', and I had thought at the time that I couldn't think of anything better. I still can't. It kind of covers everything.

Am I happy now? I don't know. No, I'm not. Not quite. It's not really possible, at the moment, and I think I have to accept that. But I am not as desperately sad as I was just a few weeks ago. And yet, there are things up ahead which I know are going to floor me, particularly as I am already in a weakened state. I shiver, and push those thoughts away. Be in the moment, I remind myself, and I sneak a look at Lizzie, who has instilled this way of thinking in me. She has her eyes closed, and the light from the flames dances across her skin. She is wearing that same poncho she had on the first time I clapped eyes on her. I am ashamed to think of the cynicism, or at least scepticism, with which I regarded Lizzie in the early days. But she soon showed us what Kate clearly already knew. She is a wonderful, wise woman, and a very warm, professional and intuitive yoga teacher.

After a while, Julie heads inside. Lizzie and I sit peacefully together, not really talking. Just basking in the heat of the fire, and the warm glow of knowing we have another successful retreat under our belts. When Julie returns, she brings with her a tray bearing mugs of hot chocolate. I take mine gratefully but at the first sip, despite its scalding heat, I shiver. "Brandy?" I ask.

"Yep! Just a little nip, to keep out the cold."

"Lovely," Lizzie beams. She raises her mug. "To the two of you."

"To the three of us," I respond. In the last vestiges of daylight, I hear a blackbird calling goodnight before it flies fast and low to the ground, right past my legs.

"Yes, Lizzie. It won't be the same without you around here—" Julie says before she's had a chance to really think about what she's saying.

Lizzie looks at her keenly. "And you?" she asks.

"I – erm…" Julie has not yet told anyone else her plans, as far as I know. Now, I think, maybe she has. Perhaps she and Lizzie have been discussing it without me. It's a silly line of thought, of course. Not helped by how unimaginably tired I am right now. A vision of home slips through my mind, and I feel my insides twist with longing. At the same time, a bat flits above us, performing lively, uneven loops, vanishing into the shadows of the trees and buildings, and then back out again. It is joined by a mate. I watch them dance across the darkening backdrop of sky while Julie tells Lizzie her plans. It seems that they have not been discussing it behind my back, then, but still I do not want to be part of this conversation. I try to focus on the bats, but I feel a sudden jolt inside me, pulling me back to earth.

"Ah, yes, that all makes sense," Lizzie says, but it doesn't feel like she's talking to us, exactly. I steal a glance at her, but she is looking at Julie. "You're right. It's right."

Childishly, I feel left out. Let down. They have plans, and I don't. I am keenly aware that they are both leaving me. In fact, the word 'betrayal' enters my head, from nowhere.

"Don't, Alice. It's not that." Lizzie puts her hand on mine. "You'll see. You'll get there."

Something about this situation, and those words, makes me feel patronised. As though they're the grown-ups, Lizzie and Julie. Seeing the bigger picture. That Amethi isn't enough for them anymore. But it's still alright for me?

I tense under Lizzie's touch, and I glare at the flames. Even though I know I should be making the most of this glorious evening, and this precious time with these people I love dearly, there is anger and resentment bubbling up in the depths of my stomach. Why is it me, staying here, left to pick up the pieces? Why am I the only one who sees the value of this place?

Why aren't I enough for them to want to stay?

Ignoring the fact that my hot chocolate is still really too hot, I gulp it down. "I think I'll go to bed, actually. I need my sleep."

There are beds made up in the smallest of our holiday cottages, which is not being used by any of our guests. The thought of the clean sheets, a comfy mattress, and uninterrupted sleep is suddenly far more enticing than a night by the fire, listening to Julie and Lizzie discuss their plans for the future, both far away from here.

"Alice…" Julie says.

"Goodnight."

As I trudge across the gravel and hear an owl calling from the line of trees, I experience another jolt – this time of regret. The rational side of me knows that I'm passing up an opportunity here, but the stubborn side of me will not allow me to go back. I head into the cottage without turning on any of the lights, and I make my way despondently up the narrow staircase, leaving the curtains open so that the night sky illuminates the room. Without even bothering to brush my teeth or get changed, I push my way under the covers, and I lie on my back, once more awash with sadness, and longing to be home, next to Holly, knowing that she is OK, and we will get through the night together.

In the morning, I shower and change and put on my best smile. After all, I still have a business to run here. The thought is at odds with what this morning is all about, but I can't help that. It's just how I feel.

Nevertheless, when I step outside, into the quiet of Amethi, I do feel a little something. I cannot deny the magic of the place, and particularly on this morning. Even so, today is not like the other summer solstice mornings. Clouds have moved in overnight, and there is a light rain in the air. It falls softly onto the gravel, and forms a fine mist on my clothing and skin. I walk around to the fire, embarrassed by my exit last night, and hoping to see Julie and Lizzie before any of the other guests arrive. When I did finally fall asleep, I slept well, and heavily, and the alarm this morning was unwelcome, to say the least. I suspect that I have only had four or five hours' sleep, but right now that's par for the course.

I round the corner to find Lizzie alone by the fire.

"Alice!" she says, warmly.

"Hi," I say. "Lovely day for it." I smile ruefully, gesturing to the sky.

"I know. Not our ideal solstice morning, eh?"

"No." I unfold a chair from under the shelter of the Mowhay, and pull it over. "Sorry."

"What are you saying sorry for?"

"Last night. I shouldn't have stormed off."

"I'd hardly call it that!" she laughs.

"Well, you know. It wasn't very gracious of me."

"You're stressed, my love. You're in shock. You're scared."

"I am," I say.

"I know. And I know it's no use saying it'll be OK. You will find that out for yourself in good time."

"I hope so. Where's Julie?"

"She ended up going in for some sleep as well. Once the drizzle began."

"Very wise."

"I don't know if she'll be out for sunrise, to be honest. I don't know if we will see it. I said I'd wake her if it clears."

"It doesn't look too hopeful."

"No. But I'm glad you're here. And it's still the solstice, sunshine or not."

There's something in that, I think, but I can't quite put my head straight this morning. I hug the words to me, though, and I smile at Lizzie. "I'll miss you."

"I'll miss you, too. But I'll be back."

"Really?" I say, my eagerness giving me away.

"To visit," she says gently. "Well, who knows? Maybe I'll

be back properly sometime, but I don't know. Whether it's with Med or not, I can feel the world calling me at the moment. I need to get back out there."

"Does that make me very dull, wanting to be in Cornwall?"

"No! Absolutely not." Lizzie pours two cups of steaming, fragrant tea from a flask. She hands one to me and I'm grateful for its warmth. "You've found your place. It doesn't mean you'll be here forever, but if you are, there's nothing wrong with that. In fact, everything about you being here feels right, doesn't it?"

"It does. But I thought it was the same for Julie, too," I say plaintively, aware I sound like Ben, or Holly.

"Well, I don't know. She loves it, I do know that. And she loves you more. When you came back here, so many moons ago, was it because she was desperate to be in Cornwall?"

"I… I think so."

"Or was it because she wanted to be with you?" Lizzie suggests. "And you were desperate to be in Cornwall?"

"I…" It's like all of that was a different life. My solitary flat; my regular, steady, uninspiring job; I was hiding away, after my horrible relationship with Geoff. But I never stopped dreaming of Cornwall. I never stopped dreaming of Sam.

"It's Julie you need to talk to about this, not me," Lizzie says, "but I've always felt like Cornwall was *your* dream. You're steady, and grounded. You know what you want, and you always have. Julie's dreams are more fluid, and she's envied you for being so sure."

"Julie's envied *me*?" I ask, astounded at such a notion.

"Yes." Lizzie says nothing more, and in fact we hear some

hushed voices, then the light from a phone half-blinds me.

"Sorry!" calls Teresa, who is on her third retreat here. "I didn't know how light it would be." She fiddles with her phone, managing to flash us with it once more before she switches the light off.

"That's OK," I smile. Lizzie has given me something to think about there, but now I need to turn my Amethi self on. And I feel a bit more like it now, anyway. I take a sip of the tea Lizzie handed me. It's strong and bittersweet. "I'm glad you could join us," I say, as Teresa and Angela and Brendan pull up chairs around the fire.

"It's getting lighter already," Lizzie says, and we turn towards the east to see that, somewhere over there, the sky looks a little less dark, and a little less cloudy. "Let's hope that it clears this way."

She pours cups of tea for the others, then suggests we do some slow, gentle yoga moves. "They won't keep us dry, but they might help us stay warm."

As the subdued morning light creeps in, a thin mist hangs around, adrift above the wildflower meadows and gravel paths. The birds begin to sing, regardless of the weather, and the day starts to take shape.

Lizzie offers a reduced version of the usual solstice ceremony by the fire, as the rain starts to fall with more fervour. We retreat into the Mowhay, where she guides us through another yoga practice, but to me it has all begun to feel a bit flat. Perhaps I'm just too tired to really get into it, but I'm glad when I can make my excuses and go.

I thank Lizzie before I leave. "For everything," I say, and I hug her.

"I have to thank you in turn, Alice. You've kept me going, you and Julie, and this place – whether you know it or not."

"I'm glad."

It feels good to have cleared the air with her, although knowing Lizzie, any ill feeling from last night would have run straight off her like the rain down the car windows.

By the time I've reached town, there is a widening patch of blue in the sky and, while I'm sorry the solstice celebrations were a wash-out, the sight still lifts my spirits slightly. I arrive to a house containing only Meg, having just missed Sam and the kids. I ruffle Meg's fur as I read the note my family have left me.

Hello Mummy, it says in Ben's sloping handwriting. *We had to go to school and work and nursry. I hop you had a good time and love you see you later xxxx*

Holly has added a wobbly 'H' and also some kisses. I check my phone and see Sam has messaged me, too:

Hope you had a good night. Holly has been great and I remembered all her stuff so no need to check! Get some sleep this morning and I'll call you at lunchtime xxxx

I don't need to be told twice. I strip off my wet clothes and put them straight in the washing machine, then I go wearily up the stairs, grabbing some joggers and a t-shirt from my drawer and pulling them on before I slip gratefully into bed, and into a deep, dreamless sleep.

15

"Sophie!" I say, as my stepdaughter wraps me in a tight embrace. "You are a real sight for sore eyes!"

"I wouldn't miss Ben's birthday," she says, spying her little brother behind me in the hallway. "How are you, Benny?"

"Sophie!" I have to step back as he flings himself at her and Holly, quickly cottoning on, comes running through from the kitchen. Sophie laughs, hugging them both.

She is so bloody grown-up these days. I refrain from making either of these observations, however. Instead, I offer her a cup of tea, and she happily accepts, following on behind with her smaller siblings practically hanging off her.

"How's life?" I ask, though I get regular updates from her. She's well into her time at uni now, and loving it all. She has no time for relationships, or so she says, much preferring to spend her time with her friends, or studying. I think she was shocked by her pregnancy scare in those Rory days, and it made her question a lot of things. I've never told Sam about that, as it never came to anything. I don't especially like keeping secrets from him, but in a way there is nothing to tell. And really, it is Sophie's secret, not mine.

As we sit at the table, Holly shows Sophie all her diabetes paraphernalia. "You do all this every day?" Sophie asks, looking at me for confirmation. I nod.

Holly lifts her t-shirt to show Sophie the tiny marks and occasional bruises made by the multiple needles over the last few weeks. As ever, it makes my stomach turn ever-so-slightly. Just the sight of that pure, soft skin, now flecked with tiny bruises and needle-prick scars.

"Well, I think you're amazing," Sophie says. "And you, too, Ben. Dad says you're doing really well at school."

I'm glad she's thought to include Ben so quickly. I am more than aware that Holly is getting a lot more attention than him these days. It's a necessity but still, he's very young to have to understand that. It's good also that it's his birthday and we can make a real fuss of him.

This year; a sign of him growing up, or so it feels, he wants only a handful of friends – all boys – and he wants to go bowling. Zinnia is also invited, along with Holly, both being more family than friends. It does mean I have to face Julie in a non-work setting, but we're muddling through, neither of us having yet mentioned my little 'episode' on the solstice eve.

Work has been flat-out and we seem to be minimising the amount of crossover time we have; I don't know that this is entirely intentional, as there is a genuine requirement for Julie to do a lot of catering at the moment, and I have also been getting in earlier, so that I can get home in time to collect Holly from nursery. I have also had to be at home for a couple of visits from the PDSN team, and I've taken Holly in for her first clinic appointment, where it felt like I was quizzed on everything, and I ended up feeling wholly inadequate and doubting that I could do what needs to be done, to take care of Holly.

Rachel called me afterwards and said that parents often feel like that: "We're just trying to make sure everything's as it should be. We are not judging you, I promise."

I appreciated the call but really, the whole thing made me feel awful. And it's like the deeper I go into this new world, the more my anger and resentment grow. I have to keep them under control for work, and at the moment that is just easier if Julie isn't there. It's sad but it's true.

Still, for the sake of Ben's birthday, and for everyone's benefit, really, I need to speak to her properly.

Once Sophie's settled down with the kids, watching *The Lorax*, I head upstairs and make the call.

It rings but goes to voicemail. I decide not to leave a message, but she'll know I called so I will hang on to my rehearsed speech until she phones back.

The only thing is, Julie doesn't call back. And when we get to the bowling alley, Luke is there with Zinnia but there is no Julie. I try not to look surprised, but Luke is clearly ahead of the game and makes sure he speaks to me as soon as he can. He's clearly trying to calm the waters, but I can't believe that she hasn't come to Ben's birthday, no matter how much of an idiot I've been.

"I'm sorry she didn't come, Alice, she just thought you might prefer her not to be here. I did tell her not to be stupid, but she's really upset."

"She's really upset?" I almost explode, in a hushed way, if that's possible. "That's a laugh."

"Alice," Luke says, with a note of warning.

"What?" I ask, fuming but having to smile and briefly

greet the parents of Ronnie, who has just joined Ben's class this year. Kids' parties are hard enough at the best of times. This is not one of them.

"Don't."

"Don't what?"

"Don't be like this."

"I'm sorry, am I being unreasonable?" I ask, knowing full well that I am, but seemingly unable to stop myself.

"You're being… you're exhausted," he says, too kind to really tell me how it is.

"Oh really? Tell me something I don't know. And while I am trying to get to grips with my little girl having a lifelong health condition, which could very well make her incredibly ill if we don't keep on top of it, my best friends are moving away, leaving the business we built up. Leaving me." I nearly sob, but I am pulled up by the sight of Ben waving me over to see the present that Ronnie has brought.

"We're not…" Luke puts his hand on my arm, but I shake it off.

"You are."

I stalk across to Ben, plastering a smile on my face and exclaiming at the lovely pirate ship bath toy. "That's lovely," I say to Ronnie's mum and dad. "Thank you so much."

And the sight of Ben's smile reminds me what this is all about. I throw myself into his party, whooping at the strikes and spares, which to be fair are not that impressive seeing as they all play with the bumpers up, and avoiding Luke as much as I can. I see him and Sam conferring at some point, and both looking my way, but rather than react, I store it up to consider later. This afternoon is not about me.

After bowling, and two of the boys being in tears at losing, there is the commiseration of a meal at the party table, topped off with jelly and ice cream. When it's time to go, I can see Luke is waiting for me, but I busy myself chatting with the other parents, until he gets the message, and he and Zinnia leave. I feel bad that I didn't say bye to her, but she won't have noticed, having had Holly's attentions all the way through the afternoon, and having been overall winner of the games of bowling.

With arms full of presents, Sam and I follow Ben and Holly to the car.

"Alright?" he asks me.

"Yep," I say, knowing full well where this is going.

"Talk later?" He's a wise man.

"Sure."

I sit through the journey home laughing at Ben's excited chatter and reliving the party. He feels very grown up, I can tell, and it's a genuine joy to behold. Holly is shattered, but her cheeks are rosy, and she looks very happy. I think for the hundredth time how lucky we are to have her, and Ben of course, but we are particularly lucky that we didn't lose her. And those 'what ifs' creep in once more: what if we hadn't found out when we did? What if she'd ended up in a coma, on a drip... or worse? I feel my heart rate speed up, as it always does. I wonder when, if ever, these thoughts will go away.

An hour or so after we get back, Mum, Dad, Karen and Ron come around for a birthday tea, bringing Ben more presents, and one or two for Holly, too. I'm pleased to see that Dad is more his old self today, and he spends a long time playing cricket with Ben and Holly, and Sam and Ron, in the back garden.

Mum, Karen, Sophie and I sit in the kitchen, drinking prosecco.

"No Julie?" Karen asks, and I wonder if Sam has told her that we've fallen out – or we would have done if we had actually exchanged any words recently.

"No," I say, taking a swig of my drink. Mum and Karen exchange glances.

"That's a shame. If it's the last time she'll get to celebrate Ben's birthday for a while," Mum says.

"Yep. Well, she was invited."

"Julie's leaving?" Sophie asks.

"Erm, yes, well, she's thinking about it. It's not common knowledge though, OK?"

"Sorry, Alice, I didn't think," says Mum.

"It's fine. Sophie's family, she should know what's going on."

"That's so sad," says Sophie.

"I know."

"What about Amethi?"

"I don't know." I really don't want to think about that right now. I don't want to think about any of it.

"Do you know if they've got any firm plans in place yet?" Mum asks. "For Toronto, I mean."

"No."

"Ah well, I'm sure it will all work out," Karen says. "One way or another."

This empty platitude sets my teeth on edge. "I'm sure it will, for them."

"And for you, love. I know it doesn't feel like it, but it will," Mum adds.

"Well, I don't see how," I hiss, not wanting Ben or Holly to hear me. "She's leaving me high and dry, she needs to sell her part of the business. I can hardly buy her out, can I? So I either sell up too, or I have to find a new partner."

This idea keeps running through my mind, of finding somebody to take Julie's place, at work at least, but I don't know who, or how that could work. She and I dreamed of our own business. We have the same ideals, or at least I thought we did. Our skillsets completely complement each other. How could I possibly find somebody else like her? Oh god, here come the tears, spilling out of my eyes and into my glass. I hurry inside, making some lame excuse. Mum follows me into the kitchen.

"It will be OK, love," she says, putting her hand on mine.

I look at her with tear-blurred vision and suddenly I have an idea. Why did I not think of this before?

"What about you, Mum? You and Dad. You could buy Julie out. It would work. We could work together, couldn't we? And you're leaving the Sail Loft anyway." My mind is racing ahead with the idea, and imagining a future working with Mum, while Dad potters about the place, doing what he used to do, keeping the gardens in order and making sure the gravel's tidy; that kind of thing, while Mum and I run the place together. Of course, we would still need a chef. Or maybe now is the chance to do things a little differently. Cut out the catering. Focus more on events and planning; maybe we could work some deals with other local businesses, to get food in when people want it. Dad could do that – like a local Deliveroo. My mum is a very professional and experienced businesswoman. She'd be perfect. My eyes are shining again, but now with excitement.

"Oh Alice," Mum says. "It's a lovely thought."

Those words alone are a kick in the teeth. I feel like I'm eight and I've just suggested to her that we get a horse and it could live in our back garden. I was sure that would work.

"But love, we've just found a bungalow we like. And we're looking to reduce our stress, not find more."

I don't say anything.

"Alice," Mum says, "I'd do anything to help you, but your dad and I need to take things easy now. I am always, always more than happy to be there for you when you need help with the kids, or anything like that. I know you've got your hands even more full now, what with Holly and everything. I want to give you a break from it all when I can, and so does your dad, but we need a break too. And we can't think about taking on another business. We're only just selling the Sail Loft."

Already, I am seeing sense and I realise it was a ridiculous and wholly unreasonable suggestion. "You've got a buyer?" I ask.

"We're in discussions, let's say that. I will tell you more, when I can. And this bungalow, Alice, it's lovely." Her face glows when she says this, and I can see how happy the thought of this new life makes her. "It's perfect, in fact."

"Well, that's great. And I'm sorry, Mum, it was a stupid idea."

"Not stupid. Optimistic, maybe," Mum smiles. "And in another lifetime, I'd have jumped at the chance to work with you. We'd make a great team, wouldn't we?"

"I think so. Or maybe we'd end up falling out, too."

"You and Julie will work it out. You always do." Mum puts her arm around me. "Now why don't you just go and put your feet up for a few minutes, eh? Everything's under control here."

I'm tempted but then here comes Ben, rampaging in with his bat under his arm, and demanding a drink. I think of Holly, and how thirsty she was before we realised that she was struggling with undiagnosed diabetes but, I tell myself, it is also very normal to just be thirsty after a game of cricket, not to mention a meal of pizza and chips. I pour him some squash, and a cup for Holly too. Mum tops up my glass and hers, and we knock them gently together.

"To the future," Mum says quietly and then, more loudly, "And to birthday boy Ben."

"To Ben!" I echo, as the others come into the kitchen and we toast our little seven-year-old, and then his sister, and then each other. I add, "To family."

16

Somehow, summer this year passes far too quickly. Sophie is with us for just a week before she's off again, travelling around France, Spain and Italy with some friends from uni, and then working at Kate and Isaac's place, to pay off the money they've lent her for her adventure. Holly finishes nursery, and we are steaming along towards her first day at school. Although as a family we are getting our heads round living with diabetes, it has cast a shadow over everything and it's a new consideration. Just when I was done with having to remember nappies, wipes, cream, change of clothes, etc., along comes something new to think about. There is no easy 'let's just go for a day out' – right now, everything needs careful consideration. Do we have needles, testing kit and strips, spare batteries, hypo treatments, etc, etc? Will we be eating when we go out – if so, what, and how will we know what the carb count is? Will we have phone signal in case of an emergency? It perhaps doesn't sound like much, but it has me on edge all the time. The fear factor has not yet gone. I hope one day it will, but perhaps it's here to stay.

I'm also up and down in the night still, and find myself immediately wide awake sometimes, for no apparent reason, in the deep darkness, and I find myself compelled to get up and check on Holly, in case some unseen force has woken me for a reason, alerting me to a problem. So far, this has not been the case. But then I feel like I have to check on Ben too. Again, so far so good. But I am living on my nerves, and it's starting to show. I have lost weight. And my eyes have that constant tiredness just behind them. Summer being summer, work is manic and shows no sign of slowing for the next few weeks. Trying to book things for people is far more difficult at this time of year, and some of our guests have been 'challenging'.

There was one group, who took over the largest of the houses. All young professionals over from London, who wanted to dine out every night, and have taxis arranged to get to and from the various restaurants. The worst of the bunch was a guy called Rupert who was just so rude and arrogant. He also, it seemed, had taken a shine to Lydia. I mentioned him to her, as he insisted on eating at the Bay Hotel a couple of nights, and was most put out on his last night, when I told him it was fully booked.

"Oh yeah, I know who you mean. He's a proper tosser. I think he thinks he's being charming. He definitely knows I'm seeing Si as well, though he's trying to pretend he doesn't. He's got that coked-up air about him, where he is pretty much oblivious to everyone else. Even if I wasn't with Si, there's no way I'd be interested."

"No, bloody hell, I wouldn't think for a minute that you would be! How is Si, anyway? Any news?"

"No, not really. He's OK, but he had to cancel his visit this week, thanks to Xavier organising some kind of publicity thing for all his clients. I'm sure he did it on

161

purpose as he knew Si was meant to be coming to see me."

"I really hope not."

"Me too. I really do wonder sometimes if this is just too much hassle. We live in such different worlds, Alice, and I genuinely don't want to hold Si back. I know that's what Xavier thinks I'm doing."

"Si's a big boy, he can make his own mind up. Anyway, it seems to me that you're being entirely reasonable – probably more than you should be."

"I don't know about that, but thank you. I knew it would be weird, having a relationship with a *celebrity* – Si hates that word – although I hadn't reckoned on quite how weird. Or the kind of pressures he's under all the time. He has to present a certain picture of himself to the world, and I can see that in Xavier's eyes I am muddying his public image."

"Ridiculous!" I huffed. "I wish I could help."

"You can."

"How?"

"Tell that Rupert bloke we're all booked up tonight."

I laughed, and I did as she asked. He was not best pleased, and suggested that if I flashed some cash, the situation might change. "I'll provide the dosh," he said, flashing his perfect white teeth at me.

"I'm truly sorry, but no amount of money will change the situation. The Bay has a set number of covers a night and they are all taken. I know the manager there always honours existing bookings. Now, I could perhaps get you into a lovely place called the Cross-Section. Amazing seafood."

"No, no, that won't do," he said. "Get me a taxi to the Bay."

"But it's fully booked…"

"We'll see."

And so I'd booked him a cab, and I messaged Lydia to pre-warn her.

Oh my god. What's with this guy? Thank you for letting me know, Alice. I'll slip off behind the scenes. Thank god we've had a walk-in party of nine, they've taken the last few seats.

I'm so sorry, I couldn't stop him.

I know, you've got to do what your guests have asked. Don't worry. He's just some spoiled little kid used to getting his own way. Not this time.

Maybe he really likes you? I felt myself grin as I tapped that message out. **This is like a romantic movie. He won't take no for an answer.**

I'm not sure that kind of thing counts as romance anymore.

No. You're right. Well stay hidden and let me know if I can help. I've told him he'll need to let me know about booking a cab back before 9pm.

Hopefully I can stay hidden till then. The team will protect me.

And they had. While the rest of Rupert's group had gone to the Cross-Section as per my suggestion, he'd taken it upon himself to head into town and to the Bay Hotel, where he'd asked for Lydia but been told she'd gone home with a migraine. He'd apparently had one drink and then headed off "with a major attitude problem" according to Tom, the head barman. As if trying to catch Lydia out, Rupert had gone back to the Bay later, and luckily she actually had headed back to her flat by then. Tom had to clear him out once all the other guests had gone, and having failed to meet the taxi I'd booked for him, he'd ended up having to walk all the way to Amethi, which is pretty dangerous along those narrow lanes in the dark.

He refused to pay for the taxi he'd missed, and he went on to complain about numerous things during his stay. In short, he was a nightmare, and the worst guest of the summer. Which I suppose means that things have improved since then.

Even so, it's not been the summer I'd anticipated, even after the year had finally begun to warm up. And I feel a little bit cheated. I read a stupid Facebook post once pointing out that you only have maybe eighteen summers with your children, and stupid or not, it's stuck in my head. I have been determined to make the most of them, but between annoying guests, slightly rubbish weather, worries about work and Julie leaving (and Julie and I not really being on the best terms), not to mention diabetes, it's felt like this one has been a wash-out. And now we're on that downward trajectory into autumn, feeling like summer never really got off the ground.

The good news is that Mum and Dad are apparently well on their way now with selling the Sail Loft, and in turn buying their new home. They have been keeping everything under wraps, which is really annoying, but also intriguing. I imagined Si and Lydia being the mystery buyers – that would make for a neat solution to lots of problems, though a premature end to Si's career. Perhaps he could make a film about it.

Another bonus is that after all the unsettled weather, we appear to be heading into an Indian Summer. Despite the nights drawing in earlier, and being distinctly chillier than just a few weeks ago, it's still a pleasure to have sunshine and heat during the day. It's put a smile on lots of people's faces; even – I'm pleased to say – mine.

17

There is a familiar feeling in the air as we step out of the house. This time of year always has such strong associations for me, as I'm sure it does for lots of people, with going back to school. There is a particular feel to it; a smell, even, and the mornings just slightly tinged with a chill which definitely was not there just a week or two ago. Leaves which were lush and green seem to have begun to curl and dry, and there are patches of pavement along the street where sycamore seeds are scattered. We had a few sycamore trees in our primary school grounds and the sight of these seeds twirling as they fall is hypnotic. I remember my friends and me throwing them into the air to watch them fall again – and splitting their sticky ends, attaching them to our noses to form little horns. I used to love the start of a school year when I was at primary school. Less so secondary, but I don't think I am alone there. Even so, it was a chance to start afresh. Maybe a new bag, or coat; a new pencil case – new stationery at the very least. There was something good about being handed fresh, blank exercise books, ready to be filled.

Today, Ben is going back, and Holly is just beginning. I feel sick and I was barely able to nibble on my toast this morning, while the two of them were their usual messy, joyful selves, spilling Cheerios and splashes of milk across the tabletop.

"Can I take a photo of you?" I ask.

Holly is not keen, but Ben persuades her. "We do it every first day," he explains. "Go on, Holly."

Always keen to please her big brother, she agrees to it, and I click away on my phone merrily, taking as many of them as I can while they are positioned in front of the house.

She does look incredibly cute in her school uniform. Julie and I used to resent our uniforms, and go to great lengths to be as creative and individual as it was possible to be. Illicit earrings, or black boots; nude nail varnish; shirts untucked. Now, I can see the good side of them. All the children being dressed the same and, most importantly, setting as level a base as possible. No worrying about what to wear, or whether your clothes are cool enough – although there were always signs. Trendy school bags and coats, or PE trainers, versus – gasp – 'unbranded' still managed to set kids apart. Not that at Holly's age this is something the children think about (although I am sure some of the parents do).

"Come on, then," I say, "let's get this show on the road."

Ben clips himself into his seat these days, though I always check he's done it right, so he clambers in one side of the car while I buckle Holly in on the other. I put their school bags on the passenger seat. Holly's is untouched and immaculate, while Ben's bears the scars and scuffs of many playground playfights and careless chuckings on the floor.

"Come on, Alice," I say under my breath. I start the car and we are on our way. As we get to the end of the road, we see Ron and Karen waving to us. They've clearly been waiting at the corner for a while. It makes me grin, it's such a lovely thing to do. I wind my window down; the back ones, too. "Good morning!"

"Don't let us hold you up," Karen says. "We just wanted to say we hope you both have a lovely day at school."

"Thank you!" Ben says. Holly stays quiet. Perhaps the nerves are catching up with her.

"Are you looking forward to it, Holly?" Karen asks.

No reply.

"You'll have a lovely time, you'll see."

"We'd better go, Karen," I say apologetically.

"Of course, you get on your way! Bye, kids!"

"Bye Granny Karen!" Ben calls, knowing she hates being called that.

"You cheeky monkey!" she smiles.

"Granny Karen!" Holly echoes and it makes us all laugh. I also feel a bit relieved.

Still, as we arrive and park around the corner from the school, I can feel the nerves closing in on me. Nevertheless, I swipe the bags from the seat, and I open Ben's door then I go round and get Holly out. She clings nervously to my hand as we walk to the school gates and even Ben seems a little bit quiet, although as soon as he sees his friends, he is off.

"Ben!" I call. "We need to go round to the reception door." He looks less than pleased at this idea.

"It's alright Alice, I'll keep an eye on him," says our old friend Becky, whose son Zach is a few days older than Ben. She and Andrew own the bar on the surfers' beach. Looking down at Holly, she says, "You look amazing! So grown up, Holly. Are you excited?"

Holly nods unsurely.

"Look how much fun you're going to have – see Ben and Zach and the others, running around? They love it here. You will too, you'll see."

I smile gratefully at her, and then walk with Holly around to the back of the school, where the small reception classroom sits slightly apart. It has a great outdoor play area, and this has been set out with lots of toys, and easels, and some ride-on cars.

"Look at that, Holly!" I am so pleased to see that she is actually beaming.

We walk to the doorway, where there are teaching assistants guiding children in smoothly, before they've really had a chance to think about what's happening.

"This is Holly," I tell Miss Burns, who I am happy to see.

"Well, Holly, I remember you from when Ben was with us! You're so grown up now. Are you going to come in? I'll show you where your peg is."

And she just goes in, my little girl. Not even a look back! I do know that it might get more difficult when it dawns on her that she has to do this EVERY DAY but today I will take this small victory. I feel a lump in my throat as I watch Holly walk inside, but I know this is a good thing. A great thing.

And the staff are primed for what to do with managing her blood sugars and injections. Rachel and I have been in to meet with them, and Rachel's done a very thorough job of explaining what everything is and does, and what to do if Holly should become ill. That part of the training is difficult to listen to. What if she becomes too confused with low blood sugars to be able to eat the sweets she needs? What if she falls unconscious?

Rachel has assured me these things are very unlikely, but even so, the stark reality of what can go wrong if we don't keep on top of it is harsh. I have to remind myself, as I often do, that so many people live with diabetes, and live well.

So this is it, I think. Holly moving on, and up, and me having to learn to trust that she will be OK without me. As I pass a mum with a crying child holding onto her for dear life, I send her a quick, sympathetic glance. Life is difficult for people in a multitude of ways. Just weeks ago, we were in hospital, terrified of what life would be like from then on. Today, my little girl walked into her first day of school with no tears, and not even a look back. I will take that as a win.

18

By the time the Amethi tenth birthday party has come around, Julie and I are on slightly easier terms, but it definitely feels like we are still treading on eggshells around each other. However, we have both recognised the need to try and find a way forward, for Amethi at least, and we are working together to do this.

"I just don't know, Alice." Julie's eyes look sore and red from spending too much time looking at a computer screen. Our accountant has sorted out our projected figures, including the hit from the hugely inflated bills we now have to pay, and we need to somehow find somebody we can convince this is a great business proposition. Or half of it, at least, if it was somebody willing and suitable to come into it as a partner. The problem is that I'm not sure either of us is convinced of that ourselves.

"I know. It's not great, is it?" I feel at turns deflated, and highly stressed. But I appreciate that Julie is as involved as she is, and not leaving me high and dry.

"Honestly? No. Unless we hike our prices up a lot, it's going to be a real struggle."

"Or run more courses?" I say, thinking of the ideas I'd had in those brief moments when I imagined Mum and Dad might be a viable answer.

"Well, yes, that would be great, but we need a replacement Lizzie, plus you'll need a chef –" I can tell she didn't really want to say this, as her eyes don't meet mine – "but that's not to say it's not doable. And there must be other writing tutors we can find. But it will take some work to arrange – and we need to know we've got the right people. *And* we need to get next year's schedule sorted sharpish, too." She says it all apologetically, and I appreciate that she's still saying 'we', but at the same time it doesn't quite ring true.

It's a real worry, all of this. In recent years, particularly since the covid pandemic began, many places have increased their prices enormously. At first this was a result of holiday-makers not being able to travel abroad and having very little choice in where they could go – it felt distinctly wrong that people were taking advantage in that way – and now the prices have stayed for the most part, perhaps inflated even further in some cases. Now, though, as people can travel easily again, coupled with the poor weather we've been having, I think Cornwall will begin to see fewer visitors. Why would people pay thousands of pounds for the chance of sitting in a damp cottage playing dog-eared board games while it tips it down outside and cabin-fever irritation grows? I'm saying this, and I love Cornwall more than anywhere on the planet! But now, to put prices down would be difficult, because of the huge increase in costs of electricity, gas, food... everything, in fact, that keeps the hospitality industry going.

Despite all of this, we have to celebrate. Everything is in place, and we have a great guest list, which includes Lydia and Si, although we are not publicising this. Shona is in charge of PR, and will put out some posts after the event, with the permission of Si (as long as his agent agrees). This might just be our – or my – saving grace, as it will bring wider, very positive, attention to Amethi.

Two people who are going to be greatly missed are Jonathan – my old colleague from the Sail Loft, who was the Amethi chef in Julie's absence, and Janie – Sam's sister. When Jon rang to say they weren't coming, I was initially a bit disappointed. Then he explained why. "Janie's pregnant!" he whispered down the phone, and I found myself whispering back, even though I was on my own.

"That's the best news!" I said. "Though I'm gutted you can't come to the party. You've been an important part of all of this, you know."

"Ah I know, we're really sad not to be there but Janie isn't feeling great with it, Alice, and I'm not sure how safe it is to fly, even though officially it's meant to be OK. It's still early days, though, so can you hold off telling anyone, please? Even Karen. She thinks Janie's got a work emergency."

"Of course, no problem." I think I understand why they haven't yet told Karen, though I feel a bit bad for her. "Thank you, Jon, for telling me. It's so good to hear something happy."

This news has helped to ensure that the smile on my face is completely genuine, as I put my best foot forward, determined that the evening will be a success. And, as Lizzie reminds me, I am allowed to actually enjoy myself. "You deserve to celebrate," she had said. "You and Julie. You've achieved a great deal here."

As ever at the moment, kind words run the risk of bringing me out in tears. "Thank you, Lizzie. You've been a huge part of it, too."

"Don't talk about it like it's in the past, Alice. It's still here. You're still here. You don't yet know how this is going to work out."

So I stand with Julie, and we greet our guests as they arrive, bringing cards and gifts and good wishes. It is not yet common knowledge that Julie is going, so to most of our guests this is the chance for a real knees-up, celebrating a successful local business.

When Lydia and Si arrive, a little ripple of whispers goes around the room, but it doesn't take long for people to settle and for the happy laughter and chatter to return to its previous volume. To some extent, people have begun to get used to seeing him around town and there is less of a buzz when he's here now.

"Hi," I kiss them both on the cheek, then I hug Lydia, taking the chance to whisper in her ear, "Things any better?"

She frowns at me and gives a little shake of her head. "Not really," she whispers, and I notice Si sending a small, worried look her way.

"I'll catch up with you later," I say, and fix a large, welcoming smile to my face, for the next guests who are just coming in. In fact, it is not hard to smile; I find I genuinely am feeling happy and proud to celebrate our ten years here.

We welcome people with glasses of locally produced wine or fruit juice, alongside platters of crudités which Julie has produced: blini with smoked salmon and cream cheese; tiny quiches with courgette and red pepper; crackers with goats cheese and a blob of chutney; crispy cubes of spicy tofu with seaweed garnish. The combination serves to ease guests into conversation with each other, and to whet the appetite for the sit-down meal – also prepared by Julie and laid out on hot dishes for people to help themselves, with mini paper cones of fish and chips, or halloumi and chips, or tofu and chips. Vats of mushy peas and jars of home-made tartare sauce; also a range of fresh salads, to try and balance out the healthiness factor. Instead of plates, we have recyclable takeaway-style cartons, which people can load up as they see fit. The guests love them and there is plenty to go around, so many come back for more.

We had originally thought we'd treat ourselves to caterers, so that Julie and I could both enjoy the evening and relax as much as possible, but with the financial situation as it is, it made sense to make use of Julie's chef skills rather than pay somebody else. It does mean we are more 'at work' than we had hoped, but I'm not sure we would have been fully relaxed anyway. It's a big evening and although it's a celebration for us, it's also a thank you to all our suppliers and a handful of regular guests who we have invited along, their names drawn from a hat. They get a free weekend at Amethi as well, the dates tying in with the autumn equinox retreat for which guests will not be arriving until Monday. Julie and I keep an eye on things and when there are more takeaway cartons on the table than in people's hands, we ask our waiters and waitresses to begin clearing away, and then we work with them to move the furniture around and clear the central space for a dance floor while, like clockwork, Half a Pint of Shanty start to set up. They put their mikes up first and test them for sound. "One, two… one, two…"

People turn round and smile, looking forward to the entertainment. But before it begins, Julie and I both have a few words to say. I'm now very glad that not a drop of alcohol has yet touched my lips. I don't think it would help the emotion of this situation.

"Can I go first?" I ask Julie and she smiles and nods. Just for a moment, it's like nothing has changed between us. I reach out and hug her, and I don't want to let go.

She prises me off her. "Go on," she says. "Just don't make me cry, OK?"

"Ladies and gentlemen," I say nervously into the mike, just about hearing my voice reverberating around the room. "Can you hear me at the back?"

"Yeah!" Paul Waters calls, with a grin. I smile, and I'm grateful to him. I immediately feel more comfortable. Shona, by his side, is whispering and pointing to her photographer, sending him up to the edge of the room, not far from where Julie and I are standing. Si and Lydia are with Shona and Paul, I note, which works very well. Neither Paul nor Shona would be starstruck by Si, both at ease with pretty much anyone and everyone.

"OK," I say, with an intake of breath. Here goes. "Firstly, Julie and I would like to thank you all for coming. It means a lot to us. And as I look around the room, I see a whole lot of people who have been instrumental in making Amethi such a success, and in making it such a wonderful place to work. I honestly feel so honoured–" I have to stop for a moment here – "to have such an amazing group of people around me. I can hardly believe that we've been doing what we do for a whole ten years. As many of you know, when we took on this place, it was almost ready to go as a group of self-catering cottages, but Julie and I wanted to do something more than that. We wanted to give guests the best kind of holiday that they could imagine – something like the catered ski chalets, but instead of in the mountains, in the snow, we wanted to do it here by the sea, in beautiful Cornwall." There is a little cheer at this. "We had no idea if it would work, but here we are. And I think it's fair to say that we still both have to pinch ourselves from time to time, to remind ourselves this is real. All of you tonight have played an important part in making Amethi a reality and I just can't thank you enough."

I stop here, as I can't find any more words. I am annoyed at myself because I've barely scratched the surface but it's all I can do to hold it together. Julie, knowing me better than I know myself sometimes, steps in, taking the mike from the stand and looking far more relaxed than I felt.

"I would like to second all of that," she says, putting her hand on mine and squeezing it. "And I would like to add something else. I'd like to thank Alice, whose incredible organisational skills are really what keep this place running. I may have the kitchen under control, but she is here every morning, taking bookings, answering questions, making sure that our guests have everything they need. She says we're partners here, and that may be true, but I say she's the managing partner. You may know that Alice and I have been friends since we were eleven years old, and I think we were probably only twelve when she first put the idea of doing something like this in my head. She used to come down here to Cornwall with her mum and dad–" she raises her glass slightly to my parents, who respond with smiles and the raising of their own glasses – "and she couldn't stop going on about it. I still have all the postcards she sent to me from her holidays down here, and later letters, telling me all about some Cornish boy or fellow holiday-maker that she'd fallen for. Sorry to break that to you, Sam!" She pauses for a moment and smiles at me. "Alice used to dream of moving down here, and she used to say that she and I would be able to run an amazing business together. I never really thought that it was more than a dream, but I know enough about Alice by now that when she wants to make something happen, it does. I know she thinks I talked her into coming back here, but what she doesn't know is I'd have gone anywhere with her, really. I just knew that for her it was always Cornwall." Julie's eyes are glistening, and I wonder where she is going with this. It seems too personal, and off-topic, given that this evening is meant to be about Amethi, not about me and her. "So anyway, once we got back down here, and Alice found Sam again, as she was always meant to do, and then when she'd mastered running the beautiful Sail Loft Hotel, I could see her looking for her next challenge. And this is where Amethi comes in. We fell in love with it as soon as we saw it, and I hope you all agree that this is a truly special place. We have been so fortunate to have ten happy years here, and to have been together through so many important times in our lives." I just hope she isn't about to announce she's leaving. Shona has cautioned against this, from a PR point of view, but it feels to me very much like Julie is wavering, emotion getting the better of her.

I catch Luke's eye and he smiles at me and gives a slight nod, so I squeeze Julie's hand and gesture towards the microphone. She looks at me, as if brought back to reality. I hadn't been planning to speak again but I think I need to step in now and round this off.

"From both of us, thank you, all of you, for being part of a truly special decade. I would love it if we could all raise our glasses now to each other, and to my beautiful friend and business partner, Julie."

"And to my beautiful friend and business partner, Alice!" Julie calls.

"And to Amethi!" shouts Lizzie, amid a lot of raising of glasses, and laughter, and general good humour. Julie and I look at each other and hug again, as we step out of the way for the band to start up. I just cannot bring myself to think about the future of this place, or my own future full stop, without Julie by my side. For now, all ill feeling has to be set aside. Tonight, we celebrate.

19

The day after the party, my head is very sore. After the speeches, I relented on my no-alcohol policy and definitely had a glass or two too many. My head is not helped by Holly launching herself at me at 6.29am, but at the same time I am just so pleased to see her happy, bouncing self, and I have to remind myself that this is a million times more important than a couple more hours' sleep. Nevertheless...

"Do you want to snuggle down with Mummy and Daddy?" I suggest hopefully, trying my hardest to hang on to the sweet oblivion of sleep.

She does her best, for all of two minutes, then, "Need a drink," she says, her panda toy tucked under her armpit. "Come on, Mummy." She is pulling at my arm.

I give in. "Alright, alright, I'm coming." I glance hopefully towards Sam, just in case he's taken pity on me, but he's dead to the world – well, he's actually snoring away so not quite dead to the world, but certainly he's not for waking.

Meg greets Holly and me at the bottom of the stairs, her tail wagging and knocking against the banister. She pads after us into the kitchen, where I put the kettle on and get a glass of squash for Holly. We check her blood sugars, which are absolutely fine. They tend to be steady first thing in the morning, as she's not eaten or been active for hours.

"TV?" I ask optimistically.

"Yes! *Milkshake!*" Holly says, bouncing with excitement at the prospect of her favourite Sunday morning TV. I, meanwhile, am not convinced I can deal with the energy levels of the eternally upbeat *Milkshake* presenters, but I will settle for lying on the settee with my eyes closed and using the power of my mind to try and block them out. I've had second thoughts about a coffee. For one thing, my stomach feels a little too delicate right now. For another, it would be like giving in to being awake. Maybe if I am very, very lucky, I can find another half-hour's sleep.

But as I close my eyes, I find I have a niggling feeling at the back of my mind. Something about last night. Oh no. What did I do? What did I say? And to whom?

I backtrack, to the band – they were fantastic. I remember dancing with Julie, and Luke and Sam, Mum and even Dad, Martin and David... oh... David. Shit.

Memory kicks in all of a sudden. I think I may have upset David. As I recall, we'd been dancing together and having a whale of a time, but then I'd... oh no, I'd started crying. Not a very professional thing to do. I remember Shona's worried face, and David shepherding me out of the Mowhay, to the office stairs, where he'd sat me down on the bottom step then sat down next to me, so we'd been squeezed in together.

"Alice... what's up?" my kindly friend asked me.

"I'm... I..." I struggled to gulp in some air. "It's Julie. She's leaving!"

"Leaving what? Leaving who? Not Luke!"

"No, no, nothing like that," I'd almost laughed at the

thought. "No, they're definitely sticking together."

I must have sounded bitter then. "Well that's good, isn't it?" David asked.

"She's leaving me!" I wailed, pathetically. "Leaving me, and leaving Amethi."

"No!" David was shocked. "Why?"

"They're going to Canada," I sobbed.

"Oh Alice." David pulled me close to him. "I'm sorry, my love. No wonder you're upset."

"I *am* upset," I acknowledged, self-pityingly.

"But she won't be doing it lightly, you know. She'll miss you as much as you miss her."

"I doubt it," I'd sniffed, well aware I sounded like a child.

"You've still got me," David said. "And Martin. I know it's not the same, but…"

An idea occurred to me then. I looked into his eyes and smiled. "You could buy Julie's share!" I said.

"I could…?"

"Of Amethi! Think about it. You're out of work, and you've got your redundancy money, and…. Hear me out," I'd said, seeing him already about to say no. "I mean, I know you'll need to see all our finances and plans and projections, but it would be amazing, working together. We'd be great. And you said you liked the idea of working in hospitality – remember, when I was in hospital with Holly, and you offered to step in." I could just see it – me and David. He's right, that it's not the same as with Julie, but after her and Sam he really is my best friend. And he's smart, and professional, and friendly. "We'd still need to find a chef," I conceded, "or else we can think about doing things differently. Cut out the catering. Or use local restaurants—"

"Alice," David interrupted me gently. "Alice. I can't."

"Oh." Cut off in full flow, I felt stunned by his immediate rejection of my idea. "Won't you even think about it?"

"No, Alice. I'm sorry. I just can't."

"Or won't. What is it with me? Nobody wants to work with me. Not Julie, not Mum, not you. You all think I'm pathetic, I know you do."

"Of course we do," he said sarcastically, his eyes flashing with irritation. Both he and I knew that was a really stupid thing to say. "Yes, Alice, we all think you're totally pathetic."

I wince at the memory. I just felt gutted, that he wouldn't even think about it. He quickly relented, softening. "Look, Alice, I really can't. And besides, Amethi is your place. Yours and Julie's. You dreamed it up together. I don't think I could ever fill Julie's shoes, and I don't really think you'd want me to."

He was right, I can see that now, but if he's right then I am left with a huge gaping hole, aren't I? Because if he can't fill Julie's shoes, who can? And if nobody can, where does that leave me?

"Don't you think we'd work well together?" I pressed.

"I think we could," he said cautiously, "but we haven't tried and tested it. And you know that joining you here would be a huge commitment. And what if it didn't work out? I would hate to lose your friendship, Alice."

"That wouldn't happen," I'd said, desperately, even though I knew I'd already lost this argument.

"We don't know that," he'd said gently.

"Fine," I'd said. "I get it."

"Alice," David had said, "don't be like that."

"I'm not being like anything," I'd said peevishly. And I'd got up and returned to the Mowhay, where Half a Pint of Shanty were in full flow. I saw Shona, with Lydia and Si, and I went to join them.

"Everything OK?" Shona asked quietly.

"Yeah, just a bit emotional," I'd smiled.

"Well as long as you're alright. If you need to talk…"

"No, I'm fine. Thanks."

"Alice, I can see you're under a huge amount of strain. Not just here but with Holly. I get it. My little brother has a whole range of health problems and I know how hard it was for Mum and Dad. Never appreciated it when I was growing up, of course, but now I do. And what with Julie—" she whispered this, although nobody would have heard her over the rousing shanty. "Look, sometimes it's just time for things to change," she said, and it somehow felt like she was talking from experience. "And it's uncomfortable for a while, and it's hard work. But that's something you and I are both good at."

For a moment, I'd thought she was going to suggest that she take over Julie's share of Amethi, but that really would make no sense. She's got a successful business of her own. I kept my mouth shut, and was glad that I did.

"So just keep your mind open and your chin up, OK, Alice?"

"OK."

"Good girl."

"Anyone want a drink?" Si had to shout above the noise of the music and the feet stomping on the floor.

"I think I've had enough," I'd smiled. "Thank you."

"Me too," said Shona. "Champagne next time though, eh?"

A bit cheeky of her, I thought, but I suppose Si can afford it.

I excused myself and went in search of David, but he and Martin had left. My apology would have to wait. In the meantime, I had to make sure that the rest of the evening was a success. That meant splashing water over my face in the toilets, a long drink of water, and a stern talking to myself. As the rest of the guests gradually drifted away into the night, I was left with Julie, Luke and Sam.

"Great night, you two," Luke said, shifting some chairs so Sam could sweep the floor where they'd been.

"Yep," Julie grinned. She'd clearly enjoyed the whole thing and was none the wiser about my uncomfortable encounter with David. To her, I suppose, she and I were back on great terms, and the whole night really had been a celebration.

I had just smiled, and said we'd better get back home to check Holly was OK. Ron had stayed home with the kids, saying he'd prefer to do that anyway, so I knew he'd have contacted us if there was any problem, but I was starting to feel worn out, and I just wanted to be in bed. Luckily, good old Brian, our age-old taxi driver, was available – he was with us before we'd finished locking up. I sat up front with him, to avoid Julie. While we'd had a good night, I still haven't got over what's happening, as proved by my childish conversation with David.

With all these thoughts of last night whirling round my head, coupled with the inane chatter of the TV presenter, I open my eyes. I reach for my phone and message my friend. I need to sort things out.

You awake? xxx

Yep. Are you? xxx

No, I'm texting you in my sleep. I need some fresh air. Want to meet at the beach? xxx

Sure xxx

Autumn is in the air as we leave the house. The leaves on the trees rustle in the friendly breeze, and I experience that brief feeling of relief that the madness of summer is over and maybe, just maybe, we can relax a little. Enjoy the comfort of warm jumpers, cosy up inside while the nights become ever longer and darker. After all these years, I know this feeling does not last, and by the time January is here I am desperate for some sunny days again, when I don't have to bundle myself and the kids up in coats, hats, gloves and scarves. But I suppose we should try to appreciate everything we can – and I know full well that Lizzie will be reminding us of this in her forthcoming Equinox retreat.

Today, though, despite the promise of cooler, stifled days, it is bright and breezy – and the sunshine bounces off the sea. I have left a note for Sam and Ben, both of whom are still asleep. This morning, just Holly and Meg and I are going out.

Meg sees our friends first and goes bounding over, full of puppylike enthusiasm. They turn and laugh, and she sits so that they can stroke her. A blast of wind from across the waves hits me and I feel immediately more awake. More alive.

"Alice!" David calls. "Hello, Holly!"

"Hi!" I smile, and go to hug him. He pulls me in close to him, and I'm so immediately glad of his warmth and capacity for forgiveness. "I'm sorry," I whisper into his ear.

"Don't be silly!" he says. "I'm sorry too."

"What have you got to be sorry for?"

"For not being more open with you."

"About what?"

The girls are already running in and out of the shallows with Meg. I can see Holly's leggings are soaked, but what does it matter?

"About what I'm actually doing, with my life and with my redundancy money."

"Well that's OK, you don't have to tell me."

"It's just been a while getting it all together. And Bea didn't want me to tell anyone, until it was definite... but even so, I should have told you."

"Bea?" I ask, wondering what she's got to do with this.

"Yes. You see... she and I are going into business together."

"Well that's wonderful!" I can't really feel jealous that David is going to start something up with his own sister. "What are you doing?"

"Well..." he pauses, weighing up his options. "You will need to speak to your mum and dad about this. But OK, we're buying the Sail Loft."

"You're not!" It makes me laugh out loud. So now I know who Mum and Dad's mystery buyers are.

"We are." He looks pleased now, having seen my reaction. "Do you think I'm mad?"

"No. Well, maybe a little. But no. I can see it now. It'll be perfect."

Those imaginings I'd had, of David running Amethi with me. I remember my words to him last night, about him wanting to work in the hospitality industry and it turns out that's exactly what he's going to do. Not with me, sadly, but with his own sister. I know straight off that it is exactly right.

"I don't know about perfect!" David smiles.

"Well, no, I'm sure there will be ups and downs. Teething problems. But you will just be so great – and Bea obviously knows it all inside-out anyway. I can't believe she's going back, though."

"She said that ever since Bob died, she's regretted giving the place up. She's never resented Phil and Sue having it," he adds hastily, "but she says it anchored her. It was the thing she did after her first marriage broke down and it kind of built her up again. But I think she also acknowledges that doing it on her own would be too much. Which is where I come in."

"And does Martin like the idea?"

"He loves it! Especially because we won't be living in. Bea will be doing that. It'll take some juggling, but now the kids are older, it should be easier to manage."

"What about the kids?"

"I think they think it means they can stay in a hotel

whenever they like!" he laughs. "They'll be disappointed. But really, it won't make a lot of difference to them. Maybe financially, at first, we won't be quite as well off, but we can more than manage. We are luckier than most."

"Maybe you can give me a job," I say, and realise I'm only half joking.

"Oh Alice, it won't come to that. Will it?"

We have stopped, and are standing side by side, looking out across the waves.

"No. Well, I don't know. The thought of working for somebody else feels quite appealing at the moment."

"But really, we won't have any positions suitable for you, Alice. It's going to be a squeeze, Bea and I earning the livings we want from the hotel."

"Oh, I know. I was joking, really. But not about the thought of being employed again. I suppose I just feel completely overwhelmed with responsibility, and even more so with Holly's situation." I immediately hate that choice of word. 'Situation' sounds like I'm tiptoeing around reality. But I also worry that I am becoming boring, mentioning diabetes every chance I get. In truth, though, I do feel an enormous weight and pressure to get things right, to not only make sure that Holly is well but that she does not feel any of the stress of it, and that we prepare the ground adequately for her to be able to go ahead and do everything all the other children can do, with as little extra fuss as possible. Along with the appointments and managing medication supplies, it is starting to feel like a job in itself.

"But you love Amethi…"

"I love Amethi with Julie being part of it. I have no idea

what it will become without her. Perhaps this is an opportunity for change for me as well."

"You mean sell up?"

"No!" Those words make my stomach lurch, and I rush to deny that is even a possibility, but I know that deep down this thought has been recurring. "I don't know. I honestly don't. I just wish somebody could sit me down and tell me what to do. It's all a mess up here," I tap my head.

David puts his arm around me.

"It'll straighten up. It will. And Sam's good, isn't he? You and he share responsibility for Holly and Ben, equally."

"He is, and we do." I'm grateful that Sam is the man he is. I've dipped into some of the online support groups for parents of diabetic children and a common complaint amongst mothers is how it's them, not the dads, that have picked up the extra duties, by default. It's the mums who take time off work for appointments, and communicate with nurseries, schools, and other activity providers. Sam is not like that. He's always been ready to take time off work if the children are ill, but somehow it's been easier for me to do it because I'm self-employed. So that is a major benefit for me of keeping Amethi. I don't have to ask anybody for time away if it's needed. But the reality is that the work won't get done in my absence. I still have to make the time for it, somehow. And some things can't wait – when there are real, live guests staying who need something immediately. I don't know. I'm starting to worry more and more about the price increases, and the slower rate of bookings for next year, which might be down to the higher cost but might equally be down to the crap weather of this summer. It will be sending people abroad even though there is the opposite problem in much of Europe, where wildfires are burning with alarming regularity.

Holly and Esme come running up. David's daughter loves being the older one, and relishes the adoration with which Holly regards her.

"Can I check Holly's blood sugar?" Esme asks. From the outset, she has been keen to help with everything diabetes. It's very sweet.

"Tell you what," I say, "let's do it together, shall we? If you don't mind, Holly?"

"I'll show Esme what to do," Holly says.

"OK," I reach into my bag, surprised. I hand Holly's kit to her and stand back as she kneels on the sand and gets out what she needs. I am ready to step in if necessary but she only needs a hand to open the test-strip wrapping. She carefully pushes it into the monitor, and she waits for the little blood-drop symbol to appear. Then she holds the finger-pricker to the pad of one of her fingers, and clicks. I feel both sick and proud at the same time, as a little spot of blood appears on the pad of her finger, and she holds the strip to it, watching the blood soak in.

She and Esme, heads together, wait for the reading.

"3.8!" Esme says, looking up at us.

"Oh, that's a little bit low," I say, but Holly is already getting herself a couple of glucose tablets out of the pouch.

"Amazing, Holly!" David says. "You're so clever!"

She beams, and I can't help but smile, too. I would not wish this on her, or on anyone, of course, but every now and then I have a flash of a positive that might come from it. I have to reach a long way to find something good about diabetes but it will hopefully help Holly be resilient – and sensitive, too. As she sits on the beach, wriggling her toes in the sand, I feel incredibly proud of my little girl and how far she has already come.

20

Before I know it, it's Lizzie's last day. Julie and I are in agreement that it needs to be special. It is the end of Equinox week, which has been a great success, and we've said goodbye to some very happy guests, who have been asking when we're releasing the programme for the next year.

"Well, we need to find a Lizzie replacement," I say, "which as you can appreciate is no mean feat. But as soon as we know what's what, we'll be emailing you all."

The truth is, we have got nowhere near finding anyone to replace Lizzie. My focus has been more on who I can find to replace Julie, while her mind has also been on the future. And while I could be mean and say she's only interested in her new life in Toronto, that would not be fair. I know she is looking ahead to that, and both stressed and excited about it, but she also is determined not to leave me in the lurch. I may be abandoned by her, but I know her well enough that I realise she will only want things to go well for me.

It is impossible, though. I'm really beginning to see that. Without Julie, there is no Amethi – either emotionally or financially. We have had the business valued and, as I already knew, I can't afford to buy her out. I'm not sure I can afford to pay the bills. Even if I could do those things, I wouldn't then be able to pay another chef and/or an admin assistant, which is one solution Julie has suggested, as a way of replacing her. I think deep down Julie knows too that it's just not viable. If I can't find somebody to fill her shoes, and become my business partner, then I think we will have to call it a day. But before I give up, I do have one option left, and I'm about to test it out.

"Julie's leaving?" Lydia asks, shocked.

"Yes," I say flatly. I've had a lot of time to (kind of) get used to this idea, and I forget how much of a shock it is to people. "But what about Amethi?"

She's got to the point faster than I'd thought she might.

"Well, exactly. What about Amethi," I say. "I'm stuffed."

"Oh, Alice. What a nightmare."

We are sitting in Joe's café, having cheese-and-onion toasties and big, steaming mugs of tea.

"It is," I say, picking at a damp sugar packet until its contents stream out and form a small heap on the table. "Although…" I look up and meet her eye.

"What?" she asks, and I see understanding dawn on her. "Me?"

"Yes," I say. "You. Well, if you'd like to. Would you?"

"Oh my god, Alice, I'm so honoured you've asked me!"

I don't want to tell her she's the third person I've approached – although now that I'm here with her, I can't believe it didn't occur to me before. It's so obvious.

"Do you like the idea?" I ask, trying not to sound too hopeful.

"Well… yes. Of course I do!"

"I appreciate you've only had about ten seconds to begin

to process it!" I laugh, heartened by her response. "So of course I don't expect you to know what you think or feel about it yet. But Lydia, I think we could work so well together. We always used to. And you've done such an amazing job at the Bay. I know we could do fantastic things at Amethi…"

"I just don't know if I'd be able to afford it, Alice," she says, gently interrupting my flow.

"Well," I say, wondering how to put this, and hoping I'm not speaking out of turn. "Is it something Si could help you with, do you think?"

Her eyes darken slightly. "I don't know about that."

"I know, I know you don't want to take handouts," I say. "But could you work it out as a loan, do you think? He must be able to afford it."

"What he can afford is not really any of your business, Alice," she says sharply.

I'm taken aback, but I realise she's right. "I'm sorry, Lydia. That was really rude of me. I'm just… I'd love for us to work together. To take Amethi somewhere new."

"I'd love that too," she says, "honestly. And I'm sorry for snapping, but I don't want to rely on Si financially. Partly because I don't want to rely on anyone but myself, ever. And partly because—" she looks around, ever mindful she may be being listened to – "I'm thinking of ending it."

"You're not?"

"I am."

"Oh no, Lydia. Why?" Of course, I already know in part why, but they're so good together. "It's not because of Xavier, is it?"

"He's just part of it. I think there is too much difference between us and how we live, to be able to make it work. Si will always be in different places, with different people. You know that week recently when he was meant to come here but didn't? When Xavier had organised that PR thing?"

"Yes," I say, remembering that pushy guest who had clearly had a thing for Lydia. I hope that she's not about to say she had her head turned by him.

"Well, it turns out that Si was with his ex that week."

"Who? Jodie?"

"Yes," she says glumly. "She's Xav's client too, and he'd organised for her and Si to do some publicity shots together. You should see them, Alice. They look so... right... together."

"That's awful," I say. "Of Xavier, I mean. And it doesn't matter what they look like together in pictures. You know that's all smoke and mirrors. I mean, I'm not saying Si's not incredibly handsome −" I am pleased to see she smiles at this − "and there's no point pretending that Jodie isn't drop-dead-gorgeous, too, but so are you, Lydia. And besides, it really isn't about that. You know that."

"I do know," she says, "and it's not really about the pictures, although they did make me feel a bit sick. But Xav's put her forward for the female lead with that film in the States as well."

"Oh," I say.

"Yes. Oh. I'm gutted. I know it doesn't mean anything. It certainly doesn't mean they'll get back together, and Si swears there is absolutely nothing between him and Jodie anymore, but she gets him, Alice. She gets his life in a way that I never will. And she's signed up for all the invasions of privacy as well, hasn't she? I haven't. I hate all that shit. So does Si, apparently, but it's him they're interested in, not me. He's the famous one. It feels very unfair that I have to keep looking over my shoulder all the time."

"Ah, Lydia," I sigh, "I'm so sorry." I am, for her and for me, but I will have to put my self-interest aside for now, and just accept that I may have exhausted all my options.

"I will think about Amethi, Alice. I'm so flattered you've asked me."

"Do," I say. "If there's any way we can do it, I'm sure we can make it work." But even as I say this, I can feel doubts beginning to crawl into my mind. Could we, really? I do love and respect Lydia enormously, but taking on a huge financial commitment together is a great risk. Still, I'll see what she comes back with. Maybe she and Si won't split up. Perhaps she will change her mind and ask him for a loan.

Whatever she decides, I feel like it is out of my hands now.

21

Back at Amethi, I am delighted to see Kate's car parked up.

I head straight over to the Mowhay, where she is sitting chatting with Lizzie.

"Hello!" I say, as she stands to hug me. "It's so good to see you!"

"You too, Alice. You've been through the mill lately," she says, looking at me sympathetically.

"It's not been the best," I laugh, not wanting to get into it. I am always close to tears these days, and I don't want them coming now. Today is, after all, about Lizzie.

On the drive back from town, I let it settle over me, that it was unlikely Lydia would be taking up my offer. After today, I will speak to Julie about putting the business up for sale. I have no idea how that will work; it's a huge thing, with an ongoing business and bookings for next year, deposits already paid, but with a mortgage and all that entails. This was not part of our dream.

"Tea, Alice?" asks Lizzie.

"Yes, please," I say, accepting the cup she offers. "That smells good."

"Equinox tea!" she smiles. "It's all about supporting change. Anyway, I need to go and check my packing, so I'll leave you two to it for a bit, if you don't mind."

"Not at all." I look at Kate. "So…" I say, as Lizzie heads off to the cottage.

"So…" Kate echoes. "How's everything going? How's Holly?"

"She's doing really well thanks," I say. "I can't believe how well she's adapted to everything."

"And you?"

"Maybe not so well," I admit ruefully.

"Yeah well, I get that. God, I'd have died if Sophie'd had anything like that happen to her."

"I know. It's been a huge shock," I say.

Kate just puts her arm around me, and I lean against her for the briefest of moments.

"But we just have to accept it. We have to get on with it," I continue.

"Easier said than done though, eh?" she murmurs, and I am just so grateful for her understanding and kindness.

"What about this place as well? Lizzie going and, if I've heard things correctly, Julie too?"

"Yes," I say glumly. "And almost certainly me as well." It's something else I will just have to learn to accept, and get on with.

"Really? There's no other way?"

"I don't know. I've exhausted all my options to find another partner, and I don't want to invite a stranger in. That could go so wrong. Maybe it's better to bow out gracefully."

"Oh, that is sad," Kate says. Again, I know she completely understands. She loves her place in Devon as much as I love Amethi. At least she is running it with her partner. Although, what would happen if they were to split up? The prospect seems unlikely. She and Isaac seem closer and stronger every time I see them.

"I just hadn't considered this might happen, which was stupid. I suppose that's a basic rule of business – have a contingency plan. And an exit plan. Julie clearly had that covered, I just didn't realise."

"I doubt it's easy for Julie, you know," Kate says gently, and this is interesting because those two have not always been the best of friends. "How are things between the two of you?"

"They've been better."

"It's a bit of a nightmare for you both, isn't it?"

"Yep."

"Don't let it ruin your friendship, though – something like that has to rise above it all. It's too precious to throw away, believe me. I've been envious of your friendship since the day we met."

"Really?"

"Yeah, of course! You know I don't find it easy to make, or keep, friends. I remember you telling me how you'd known each other since school. I barely had any friends while I was at school and certainly nobody's bothered to keep in touch since then. That first time we went out, and I kept pressing you to do it again, I cringe when I think of how I was then! But I was so desperate for you and me to be friends, Alice. I thought that as Julie was seeing Luke, and you were annoyed at her, maybe I could take her place."

I do remember what she was like; the text messages and the abrupt responses if I turned down an invite. Poor Kate, she was a lonely single mum. Little did I know that the ex she used to talk about missing was Sam. What a strange, small world it can be.

Kate is right about me being annoyed at Julie back then as well. She had not long split up with Gabe, and Luke was clearly in a vulnerable position with his mum being ill. But maybe more than that, if I'm honest, I felt my nose put out of joint because she and I had come down here together, and she wasn't spending enough time with me – in my opinion. And now I'm annoyed at her all over again, for living her life and making her own decisions; this time with Luke and Zinnia firmly at the heart of them. Perhaps I am more of a needy friend than I like to think.

Kate continues, thinking again of Amethi, "Just because Julie's moving on, does it really have to mean you need to do the same? Could you borrow money from the bank, to take the whole place on? Then you don't need to find another partner."

"I've thought about it. Looked at the numbers. I don't know, I think it's just too much."

"Well, whatever happens, you and Julie have done incredibly well to keep it going so brilliantly, for so long," Kate says. "You should always feel proud of what you've achieved here."

"Thank you. I do appreciate that, and I know you're right. And I am trying to convince myself that with things as they are, with the rising costs of… well, of everything… maybe it's not such a bad time to look to do something new. The problem is, I have no idea what."

"It'll come good," says Lizzie, swanning back into the room.

"I hope so," I put a smile on my face, remembering that today is about Lizzie, not me. I also realise that Julie will be here in a moment, and I do not want to be talking about this when she comes in. "Now come on, let's get the outside table set, and we can have lunch."

"Perfect!" says Kate. She helps me take out the table covering, plates, cutlery, and a vase of flowers from the Amethi garden. Julie comes out with a glass jug of water, ice cubes bobbing around amongst slices of cucumber and sprigs of mint.

"Do you mind helping me bring out the food, Alice?" she asks, so politely it hurts more than it would if she'd actually been rude.

"Of course."

I follow her into the kitchen, as I have so many times over the years, and let her give me instructions of what to get, and from where. Normally, we'd be laughing and joking, but there is none of that today. I want to tell her I'm sorry, but I don't even know where to begin.

Instead, I follow her instructions and take out a loaf of still-warm granary bread, on a wooden board, and a block of creamy Cornish butter. Julie brings a couple of bowls of salad, and then we go back in for the cheese and olives.

I'm sweating as I get back to the table. "We've lucked out with the weather," I say. "There won't be many more days this year we can be sitting outside like this." My negative mind flicks to the thought that this might actually be the last time we do this, ever. That, depending on when we find a buyer, this all could be out of our hands by the time the weather's warmed up next year.

I give myself a stern talking to. What will be will be. I have to just think like that. And I have to turn my mind to Lizzie, and making sure she has a happy and memorable last day before she goes on her travels.

As we tuck into the food, we begin to relax, and take turns sharing the memories we have of this place. Some funny, some emotional. Julie risks mentioning the time that Tony stayed with us – the guy who turned out to be my online troll, and erstwhile friend of my long-ago, controlling ex.

I mock-shudder. "That was scary."

"And infuriating!" Julie adds. "Remember those reviews he was leaving? They could have had us dead in the water before we'd even got off the ground, to mix my metaphors."

Lizzie takes us back to the snowy Christmas nearly five years ago, when she'd supported me through Holly's birth. That has all of us in tears – although Kate was not here for it, she is a sensitive soul and moved by the tale, despite having heard it all before.

Kate talks about how much she'd loved working here, and how Amethi had helped inspire her own decision to start the business with Isaac. "Far enough away that we wouldn't be in competition!" she smiles.

"Remember when we thought the Bay Hotel was after our business?" Julie asks, nudging me.

"Oh god, yes, I do. All of these things seem so long ago," I say wistfully. "And yet like they were just yesterday."

"Life's like that," Lizzie says. "And the mind. Memory. It's not all linear. I know that even years from now, there'll be times I find myself back at Amethi. We all will," she says surely. "To

Amethi," she says, raising her glass. "No matter what the future brings, it won't change what has already been."

It's classic Lizzie – obvious, but no less true for being so. And it does have Julie and I shooting a look, and even a grin, at each other, which I suppose is progress. I mouth: "Present?" Julie nods.

"Lizzie," I say, as Julie stands to head inside, "we have a little something for you which I hope will come in useful on your travels."

Julie returns, bearing a very large paper bag – Lizzie would not approve of unnecessary wrapping. She looks like she is about to cry as Julie hands the gift to her.

"Oh!" Lizzie says, pulling the large rucksack out. "Oh my god, this is amazing!"

"Well, we know you don't really like brand-new things," Julie said, "but on this occasion we thought we'd better get something to start you off with. It can get battered and worn over the years and help tell your tale. And," she says, pulling an envelope out of her pocket, "we thought we'd help you get that story off to a start."

Lizzie opens the envelope to find a woven badge decorated with a picture of Amethi. She sobs, and Kate puts an arm around her.

"This is too much," she says. "So brilliant. I will treasure it. And I feel completely spoiled with this shiny new rucksack!" She laughs through her tears. "I would never have got myself something like this. I mean, because, of the expense, not because I don't like it…"

"We know what you mean!" I laugh too. "Think of it as your home on your back."

"Like a snail," says Kate.

"Or a Teenage Mutant Ninja Turtle," suggests Julie.

The mood lightens and brightens, and we take a walk together around the grounds, noting how the majority of flowers have gone now; just the late bloomers remain. But the leaves cling stubbornly to the branches of the trees, and the birds are still in full song. For a moment, I feel like there is a hint of spring in the air. A whiff of a promise. But, I remind myself, this is autumn. We are approaching an end, not a beginning.

"There will always be a part of me here," Lizzie says, as the four of us stand between the trees and the field, looking back towards Amethi.

She puts an arm around me, and an arm around Julie. I put my spare arm around Kate, on my other side.

"The year's turning," Lizzie says.

And everything's still up in the air, I think, but I say nothing. Just take a breath, and close my eyes for a moment. When I open them again, I watch the congregation of house martins, swifts and swallows high above, readying themselves for their long, arduous migration. Above the yellowy-brown wildflower field, the tall grasses still standing but readying themselves to fall, flits a beautiful emperor butterfly. It flutters towards us, then heads high into the air, back across the field and over the hedgerow. I watch its progress until I can't tell whether I can still really see it, or if I am merely imagining that I can.

22

With Lizzie gone, it feels already like things have started to change at Amethi. Although she didn't work here full time, since she moved into the little cottage, which was once my home, she has been a constant, comforting, calm presence. I decide to face the music and take Kate's advice, and make things right with Julie. Of course our relationship is the most important thing; ironically, that's why I'm so put out, and why I'm acting up. It hurts, so much, that she is going away. But I know that she must, that it's the right thing for her and her family.

"Coffee?" I ask, when she arrives on Monday lunchtime.

"Erm… yes please," she says, giving me a look that she thinks I haven't noticed. It used to be commonplace that I'd offer her a drink as soon as she got here, and we'd talk through work things before we'd go our separate ways and get on with our days. Lately, this has been rare.

We head into the kitchen together and she fills the kettle while I rinse out a cafetière. I have already drunk far too much coffee today, but not to worry. My hands feel cold, and my eyes are sore, from sitting in front of the computer for too long. I need something hot and bitter to sort me out.

I almost want to say this to Julie because I would put money on her saying, "Hot and bitter, like your men," and us both snorting with laughter. But I am not ready to joke yet.

Once the coffee is ready and the milk is warmed, we take a mug each and go through to the Mowhay. It reminds me of sitting here when Lizzie came to break her news. The year has fully turned since then. Outside, the leaves are just beginning to reveal their autumn colours and the flowerbeds, cleared over the weekend by Dad, look sparse, ready for their winter rest. When they next raise their heads, who knows what life will be like here? What I want to talk to Julie about may have some bearing on that.

"What if we just sell out?" I say, not wanting to beat around the bush.

"Sell up?" she asks.

"Well yes, but I do mean sell out as well."

"You don't mean…?"

"I do."

Unspoken is the name of the luxury holiday company that has been buying up places in and around the town over recent years. The owners don't live in Cornwall – or even in the UK – but they have agents locally who are always scouting for new places to refurbish (painting walls white and knocking down walls where they can, for the 'ultimate in open plan living') and upgrade (this usually means adding a hot tub).

"But we hate them!"

"Hate's a strong word, Julie."

She looks at me sharply, and sees I am smiling. She looks relieved. "So we do still hate them?"

"Yes of course we do. But I just don't know how many other options we have. I mean, with no Lizzie or Lizzie-

207

replacement, the yoga's gone. With no Julie or Julie-replacement, the catering's gone. It will never be the same again, but we have had ten amazing years. I don't like the idea of selling to them any more than you do, but perhaps Amethi is not so much this place but a state of mind."

Again, I am smiling, and this time both of us dissolve into laughter.

"Oh Alice, I've missed this."

"Me too. I hate it, being at odds with you."

"But you are odd."

"Look who's talking."

I'd discussed it with Sam over the weekend – what it would mean for us, if Julie and I sell out, as I will insist on calling it. The company I want to approach may be a bit different to us, but they have largely glowing reviews from their guests, and I know that financially they will be more than able to afford to buy us out. I also happen to know that Paul Waters is mates with the business owners, and I can ask him if he'll put us in touch. Hopefully with that link they won't try too hard to knock the price down.

"But what about you, Alice? What are you going to do?"

"I don't know yet. I think first of all we need to work out what to do with Amethi. Julie and Luke want to go in a few months' time. I want to know what we are doing before they go, even if it's not all signed and sealed before then."

"But Amethi was your dream."

"It was. But I think it's had its day."

"I can't believe I'm hearing you say that." Sam had looked concerned.

"No – neither can I, really, but life moves on, doesn't it? We have to roll with things sometimes and then work out how to make them better. And honestly, the more that time goes on and I consider the implications of everything running a business means – on top of caring for Holly, and for Ben of course – I just feel like I can't do anything as well as I want to. And I don't like that feeling."

"OK. Well, you know I'll support you, and we'll find a way to manage. See what Julie thinks." He had kissed me, and leant his forehead against mine.

"Thank you, Sam. You don't know how much strength I draw from you."

"I do, Alice," he murmured. "Because I get the same from you. We're strong together, aren't we?"

I circled my arms around his waist and drew myself towards him. Idealistic and clichéd though it may sound, I really do feel like I'm beginning to see the true value in things, and recognise what is most important in life. I will never give up work, and what I do will always be incredibly important to me, but there is nothing – nothing – that could be more valuable than the relationships I have with the people that I love.

"I suppose it can't hurt to just put the idea out there," Julie muses now.

"That's what I'm thinking. It's not like we'll be committing to anything."

"Okay," Julie sighs. "Hot tubs it is."

"I think if they do take over, they'll do something great with the place. I mean, not greater than what we've done, but they're pretty good at making their properties special. I can imagine a playground or something—"

"In place of the wildflower meadows?"

"I don't know. I hope not. But maybe. I think the thing is that if we're going to sell, we have to accept it just won't be ours anymore."

I don't want to say what I'm thinking, but she vocalises it instead: "I know, I can't really say what should and shouldn't be, seeing as I'm the one that's set all this in motion."

I just smile.

"Smug," she tries tentatively.

"Says the person moving to Canada!"

And that's it. There's a tangible sense of relief and it feels as though, in agreeing on a possible solution, we have come back together.

"To selling out," I suggest, raising my mug.

"To selling out."

I waste no time in getting in touch with Paul, who says he will happily make an introduction.

"Also, Shona and I have been meaning to invite you and Sam over," he says. "Fancy Sunday dinner at ours soon?"

"That would be great, thank you. Could we hang on till after you-know-what though, please?"

Julie is nowhere near, but I still feel like I have to whisper and use rather rubbish code when referring to the forthcoming party.

"Of course. That should give Shona time to get things sorted, too," he says.

"Sorted?" I ask.

"Oh yeah, she's just a bit busy with work at the moment," he says vaguely.

"When isn't she?"

"Too right," he says. "Anyway, I'd better crack on, but I'll drop Peter a line later. OK if I pass on your mobile number?"

"Of course. Thank you, Paul." It hasn't escaped my attention that it was Paul who helped ensure that we got Amethi, and now it looks like he might be helping us sell up. I suppose it's kind of neat, in a way. Even so, once I've hung up, I feel a bit sad, that the end of it all is becoming reality.

And it doesn't take long for Peter to get in touch, which I assume is a positive sign. We arrange a Zoom meeting with Julie and with his partner, Andrea, and in the meantime I agree to send him over the information he asks for, including the valuation we've had on the buildings and business, as well as the bookings we've in place over the next year, and a potted history of Amethi.

"It sounds like you've put your heart and soul into this place, Alice," he says.

"I suppose I have. We have," I correct myself.

"Well, send it all over, and I'll have a look to see if it's something we want to consider. And if we should, eventually, end up taking it on, you can rest assured it will be in good hands. Our holiday-makers love our places, and we're rated 4.8 stars on customer service."

It makes me feel a little bit better. But only a little bit.

In the meantime, all is going ahead with Bea and David's purchase of the Sail Loft and, in turn, Mum and Dad getting their dream bungalow. In honesty, I don't think that a bungalow was their dream, but when I finally get to see it in real life, I can completely understand why they had set their hearts on it. Set back from the street, surrounded by lawns and flourishing flowerbeds, and with a view of the sea from the large picture window in the lounge, it is quiet and secluded. Yet just along the road is a row of shops, and a bus stop, and a little further down, towards the beach, is the train station.

It's clearly been beautifully looked after, and the carpets and floors are spotless. I cast my eyes about for signs of damp, and see none. The sunshine falls appealingly through the wide windows of the kitchen, across the work surfaces. I can already picture Mum and Dad here, and us coming for visits. It feels very much like a home – in a way that the Sail Loft, love it as I do, never really could.

"It's really well insulated," Mum gushes, "so we'll be cosy in the winter, and your dad already has plans for the garden."

"As long as he doesn't overdo it," I say.

"Yes, he knows that. I've made it quite clear that he will have to take lots of regular breaks, especially if he wants to carry on with his town council work."

"Will he be allowed to, if he doesn't live in town anymore?"

"That's a good point!" she laughs. "But I think that moving three miles away, we'll be just about considered local still."

"You'd be surprised," I grin. "What about you, Mum? I don't want you getting bored."

"Oh, no chance of that. I want to help you more, with the children, if you'd like me to."

"Well of course, although actually I may also be a lady of leisure, for a while." I explain to her what we are considering for Amethi and I can see she's not one hundred per cent convinced, but she is also a realist and understands that this is the way things have to go sometimes.

"I wish I had been able to do it," she says.

"Do what?"

"Go into business with you."

"No, Mum, honestly, don't give it a second thought. It would have been completely the wrong thing to do. You were right to say no."

"But even so, I hate to see everything you've worked so hard for going to waste…"

"It's not going to waste, I promise. I think perhaps things like this are meant for only a finite amount of time. Like you and the Sail Loft. You work hard at it for the future, but more for the present. Who knows what might come next for me?" I say with more confidence than I feel.

"Oh Alice," she says, and hugs me. Then, eyes shining as she surveys her new home: "Do you really like it here?"

"Yes, Mum. I really do."

23

In the week leading up to Julie and Luke's party, I am a bag of nerves. I'm so glad that it's being held at the Bay, not at Amethi. Even so, I'm responsible for all the details. Lydia is happy to help, her staff taking deliveries of food and drink, but making sure that everything is in place is up to me.

I go through my list multiple times a day, and I am pretty sure that everything's OK, and that I know the guest list inside-out.

Sam has told Julie and Luke that we are taking them out for the evening, and that Karen and Ron will have all three children with them. At the moment, none of the children have any idea about the party, as it was too much to expect them to keep such a secret. Karen suggested that they have the kids all afternoon, and that way she can help them get ready. I've bought Zinnia a dress that I think she will like, and I've bought Holly a different colour in the same style, as I know she'll happily put on anything that Zinnia is wearing. Ben has a polo shirt and shorts – the closest I'd be able to get him to wearing something smart.

"So where are we going?" Julie asks me for the thirtieth time today.

"Julie, if you can't remember, I'm not going to tell you again." I grin. It feels so good to be back on our normal terms. We are a team once more, and well into discussions with Peter and Andrea about them taking Amethi into their 'portfolio', as they call it. That in itself is stressful so with trying to keep on top of things for the party, I am feeling like my head might implode. Or explode. One of the two.

On Friday night, I can't sleep. Trying not to disturb Sam, I lie in bed, the same train of thoughts running round and round my head, accompanied by an annoying song that I heard on the radio earlier. Every now and then, it seems that I nearly fall asleep, but my brain kicks in and catches me just in time – as if to say, "Phew, that was close. Nearly dropped off then."

I also still have to do a full day's work first, with a new tranche of guests arriving, so by the time Sunday comes around, I am going to be well and truly wiped out, but we have a clear day then and I'm hoping for lying on the settee and watching films, possibly with a large bar of Dairy Milk.

I do eventually find some sleep, and when my alarm goes off, it is very, very hard to wake up. I am dangerously close to using the snooze button on my alarm. Then I remember what day it is, and my eyes spring open.

"Alright?" Sam asks.

"Yes," I say. "I think so. Sorry, did I wake you?"

"No, I've been up a while."

"Are you OK?" I ask.

"Yeah... well, kind of." He looks sad.

"Thinking about Luke going?" I ask, shuffling closer to him and putting my arm across his waist.

"Yes, that. And thinking about Holly, too. I don't know... I feel like it's only just hitting me now. Like those first few weeks were all about survival, and learning how to do everything. Now I'm seeing the future, and it's properly dawning on me that all of this stuff is forever."

"I know," I say, not really wanting to talk about it now, but knowing I have to. Sometimes the only way I can get things done is by compartmentalising everything, and today is already so full, I haven't allowed space for contemplating this stuff. But Sam needs to talk, so I need to listen.

"I keep wondering if it's something we've done – and I know, I know it's not. Or at least not as far as anybody knows. But she's so little, Alice." I can hear tears in his voice. "And do you know what Steve's wife said to me the other day? That it's probably good she's got it now, as she won't know anything else. I could have swung for her. Honestly, I know she meant well, but really, am I meant to feel pleased that she's got to live with this shit for nearly her whole life?"

"I know," I say. "I've heard that one, too. If people really thought about it, they might not come out with things like that. But I'm sure they're all coming from a good place."

"Yes, and we end up having to just have to swallow it and make them feel alright about it too."

"I was looking through one of those Facebook groups, and someone had posted that their kid doesn't get invited to as many things, or even round to friends' houses, even when they've had other kids at theirs. Lots of people commented that they've had the same experience. People saying their kids are missed out of sleepovers. As if they need to be made to feel any more different!" I exclaim angrily. "I mean, I suppose I get it – it's a bit of an unknown, and maybe a bit scary. To be fair, I didn't understand anything about diabetes a few months ago either. But I like to think that I wouldn't just drop somebody. I hope I'd want to learn how to support them. It's made me realise even more just how lucky we are to have Julie and Luke. They've been there from the very start, Julie doing all those meals for us. Having Holly and Ben over as normal. Learning how to do it all. Shit, Sam, what are we going to do without them?"

"I don't know," he says sadly, sliding his arm around me and rubbing my shoulder. "I really don't."

We allow ourselves a few minutes of wallowing in our grief – because that really is what it is. But we cannot wallow for long, and Sam knows it.

"We'll be OK, Alice."

"Of course we will," I say determinedly. It hits me that Sam has been so supportive to me lately, I haven't given enough thought to how much all of this is impacting him as well. "We will be more than OK. We'll be great. Amazing!"

It makes him laugh, as I am hoping it will, and I sit up and kiss him.

"Go on," he says, "go and have a shower and I'll go downstairs and put the kettle on."

"Thank you. I am going to need gallons of coffee to get through today."

"Your wish is my command."

Sam not only makes coffee, but pancakes too, and I come downstairs to find Ben and Holly sitting at the kitchen table, waiting impatiently.

"Mummy first," says Sam. "She's got to go to work."

I sit with them for ten minutes, knowing it's important to

stop for just a short while, even though I am itching to get to Amethi. At least Julie isn't coming in today. It means that I am free to deal with any last-minute problems that might occur, without alerting her.

Thankfully, there are very few issues. Skaburst get stuck on the motorway for a while, which causes a mild panic, but thankfully they have set off in plenty of time, and still arrive in town by mid-afternoon. They are staying at the Bay, so they are all sorted, and Lydia messages to say what a great bunch of people they are.

The new groups of Amethi guests arrive within just over an hour of each other. There are only three lots of people this week, including one large party, which I am slightly surprised to see includes that Rupert bloke from earlier in the year – the one who'd taken an interest in Lydia. I open their booking and see that they have filled in the form with just initials and surnames, which I suppose is why I hadn't picked up on it before. I greet them as I would any other group, and I suppose I should be grateful to him for coming back, and bringing more friends with him. I've booked them into a harbourside restaurant in town this evening. I just hope he stays clear of Lydia this time, especially as Si is here this weekend.

With everything in hand at Amethi, I go home to get changed. Karen and Ron have kindly agreed to bring all three children with them, as Sam and I need to get to the Bay early, to make sure everything is ready, and to greet people as they begin to arrive.

Sam is then set to go and collect Julie and Luke, and give

them some flannel about why I'm not with him.

Exactly how to spring the surprise on them has been giving us some trouble. Images of TV-show surprise parties kept insinuating themselves, with all the guests hiding and jumping out, shouting "Surprise!" Which really is a bit unnecessary, really. In the end, we decided it would just be enough for Sam to bring them here and them to walk in and see everyone. But I absolutely, one hundred per cent, need to be at the door when they arrive.

Lydia, of course, is managing everything beautifully. She has fed the band, and she calls through to one of their rooms so they can come and say hello. They have their set list sorted, so that is one big item ticked off the list.

The main function room, with the huge window looking out to sea, is decked out with twinkling lights, and there is a big interchangeable lettering board, similar to the old-style cinema signs, which tonight reads: 'WELCOME, LUKE & JULIE. HAPPY 10TH ANNIVERSARY'. The chairs are wrapped with bows, as they would be for a wedding, and each table has bowls of wrapped chocolates, from which guests can help themselves. Anything like this now makes me think of Holly. While before I wouldn't exactly want her taking handfuls of sweets – she is only four, after all – I would have been fairly relaxed about it at a party. Now, she can hardly have an injection every time she wants to have a sweet or two. I have pre-empted this, though, and brought her a bag of snacks which are low-carb and, with the amount of running around she is likely to be doing this evening, I think she will be able to get away with one or two sweets if she really wants them. Apparently, according to

Rachel, if she has an insulin pump, this kind of thing will get easier, but I don't know if we are ready for that yet. Selfishly, I find it hard to accept the thought of my little girl living with something permanently attached to her via a cannula. But if it does make life easier, I think we'll have a proper look at it soon.

For now, though, I need to focus on this party. I run through everything with Lydia. Food and drinks are perfect, and the Bay are supplying all glasses, crockery, cutlery, etc. All is laid out beautifully, including trays of glasses which will be filled just before guests are due to arrive. Tick.

Drinks on arrival, and then Sam will go and collect Julie and Luke. When they get here, we need to give them time to wander around and chat to people. This will be followed by a buffet, a speech (maybe 'speech' is too grand a word) from me, and then the bar will open, and the band will play.

Mum and Dad are the first to arrive, and come in with a gift bag for the happy couple. Damn! I hadn't thought of this. Lydia smoothly gets a couple of her staff to bring in a spare table, and that's that sorted.

"Can we help with anything?" Mum asks.

"No thanks, Mum. Tonight is all about relaxing and enjoying yourselves. Get yourselves a drink and find a seat. Maybe that big table near the window, then Karen and Ron and the kids can join you when they arrive."

Next in are Bea with David, Martin and their two. They look incredibly happy – well, the adults do; the two kids are busy looking at their phones, although they do each give me a smile and a hug.

"How's it going for Tyler this year?" I ask quietly.

"So much better," says Martin. "They've moved things around a bit, so he's not with that kid anymore. He seems much more settled, and focused."

"That's brilliant news. I'm so pleased. Help yourselves to drinks and head on over to Mum and Dad if you'd like to, there's plenty of room at their table."

Next are Julie's mum and brother, who are staying at a little cottage down the street, and then Karen, Ron, Zinnia, Holly and Ben. They are full of excitement, and Zinnia is very proud that this is all for her mum and dad.

"You look beautiful!" I kiss her. "They're going to be super excited to see you here."

"Holly OK?" I can't help asking Karen, quietly.

"Of course," she says. "She did have a hypo this afternoon, but we coped, and we did her injection with her tea as well."

"You are amazing!" I say, hugging her and feeling the excitement of the evening flowing into me.

The room is soon filling up, and Si has skulked in, I notice, joining Paul and Shona, who are seated not far from Mum and Dad.

Sam has messaged to say he's on his way back, and I'm pacing impatiently near the door. To avoid anyone trying to engage me in conversation, and me missing Julie and Luke's arrival, I step outside. Next week, the clocks will go back, and it will be properly dark at this time. As it is, there are a few last scraps of light in the sky. The gulls call from the rooftops, to each other and perhaps just for the hell of it, while to the other side of the building, the sea blusters against the rocks.

A few people wander by while I wait: an elderly couple, and a group of people in their late twenties/early thirties. It takes me a moment to recognise them as Rupert and his fellow guests from Amethi. I bow my head, hoping that they don't recognise me, but they are too tied up in their own conversation to notice me.

"You are an idiot, Zed!" I hear one of the women say loudly, bumping into her companion.

I don't have time to think about them anymore, as here is our car – and here are Luke and Julie, clambering out and grinning as they greet me, still none the wiser as to exactly what is going on. Sam goes to park, and we wait for him to return.

"We're eating at the Bay!" Julie says, nudging Luke. "You're dressed up," she says, assessing me and then twirling around, asking, "Will I do?"

As ever, she looks more than beautiful, and I tell her so.

"Sorry, I'm taken," she says, and links her arm through Luke's, kissing him on the cheek. When Sam reaches us, I take his hand, and we lead the way inside, and stand back to watch Julie and Luke's faces as it dawns on them what is really going on.

"No!" Julie gasps, while Luke stays quiet, his face melting into a huge grin. They look around, and begin to recognise individual people, exclaiming and waving.

"Happy anniversary," I say.

At the same time, they both sweep me into a huge hug and by the time they let go, we're all crying. Sam gets the same treatment.

"This is all down to Alice," he says. "Don't thank me."

"Oh my god, Alice," says Julie. "Thank you so much. Really. I can't tell you how special this is."

"You deserve it. Ten years!" I say.

"I know. It makes me feel old, thinking I've been married that long."

"You are old."

It makes her laugh, but I can see she is shaking with emotion.

Lydia comes over, offers them her congratulations and hands them each a glass of champagne. "Go and have a wander around and greet your subjects!" she says, and they do. I stand back for a moment, so happy that everything so far has gone as it should. Holly comes up for a cuddle and I lift her into the air, her arms around me. She feels heavier than she did a few months ago, and I know she is taller, and that can only be a good thing.

Meanwhile, Ben and Zinnia dart around the room, chasing each other between groups of adults, and keeping an eye on the food table. Before long, it's time to take off the covers, and there is soon a line of people snaking towards the pile of plates. I usher Julie and Luke to the front.

"Come on, make sure you get first pick!" I say.

"Only if you join us," says Luke, handing me a plate.

"I am quite hungry," I muse.

"I'm not surprised!"

We load up our plates and head over to Mum and Dad's table. I'm pleased to see them both looking relaxed and happy. Bea is filling them in on the redecorating that she and David are planning at the Sail Loft in January when it's quiet – "Not because we don't like it as it is, but to make it ours. Mine and David's – it's extra important, because it's been mine before, and I need to know that he feels it is just as much his."

"I completely understand," says Mum. "It is such a special place, Bea, and I just feel honoured that we've been able to be its caretakers for a few years."

"It's been a real joy," agrees Dad.

Sam joins us, ushering over the kids, who have wasted no time in filling their plates, even though they've already had tea.

All around the room, people are sitting and chatting, eating and drinking. It feels like a truly happy place and a truly happy evening.

As the food is consumed and the plates cleared away, I take the microphone. My knees feel like jelly as the room hushes with quiet expectation.

As I clear my throat, I catch sight of Julie's mum, Cherry, who gives me a huge smile. She already has tears in her eyes. I return the smile and search out Julie and Luke. They look at me, and then at each other, and Luke puts his arm around Julie's shoulder.

"Good evening everyone," I begin shakily. "And thank you all for coming. Thank you also for managing to keep this secret for so long!" This is an easy line to get a little light laughter going, and make everyone feel good that they have been part of the surprise. I continue. "Ten years is a long time. A decade. It seems significant, so much that we measure our time and our fashions in decades. The nineties, for instance – that was the best one–" a little more laughter helps me relax into this – "and I was thinking about what we would say typifies this first decade of Julie and Luke's marriage. First and foremost – parenthood. They have beautiful Zinnia, who shapes their lives together, and makes them smile every day." I see Zinnia creeping closer to Luke, and nestling into his leg, smiling shyly. "Next, is travel. They've had time living in India, and Luke has been back and forth to London a lot, but even when he's away, the three of them are still so together." I decide it's best not to mention Canada, although I think most, if not all, people here must know about it by now. "Hard work. Luke, with the business he's built himself and made into such a success; Julie, my partner at Amethi." *Deep breath, Alice.* "In fact, Luke, I hope you don't mind me focusing on Julie just for a moment, but she has helped me make dreams come true in my life. From stopping me buying sweets so I could save up for the Cure album I wanted, to persuading me to move down here, and then agreeing to be my business partner. I couldn't ask for a better friend, and I love her to bits."

I glance at Julie and see she is gazing at me with glossy eyes. She raises her glass in a silent toast. "And love. That's the key ingredient of this last decade. Julie and Luke love each other, clearly, and they love Zinnia beyond words. They love their friends, their families, they love work, and they love life. It's not always easy–" I don't mention Jim or May but I meet Luke's eye here and I hope he knows I'm thinking of them – "but Julie and Luke also love a challenge. Sometimes challenges come unbidden but it's clear that these two will face them head-on, with positivity and humour, and together. This is part of what makes them so perfect for each other. I can't wait to see what the next decade will bring. To Julie and Luke, everybody."

As the guests raise their glasses, Julie and Luke come towards me and envelop me in a huge hug. We are all crying and I realise the mike is still on. I laugh, and try to put it back in its cradle, but Julie takes it from me.

"I just want to say," she stops, and has to blow her nose. It makes everybody laugh. "Sorry about that! I just want to say, how very grateful we are to all of you for coming tonight. It feels very decadent – fittingly, given the word – to be celebrating ten years of married life. And I can promise you that this evening has come as a genuine surprise to us both. But what a treat, to be able to stop and look back, and mark this occasion with you all. I can't believe she's managed to keep all this from me, but I would like to say such a huge thank you to Alice, for arranging this, and for thinking of it in the first place. As you all know, Alice and I go back years and we've also just celebrated a decade at Amethi. I'm sure most of you also know by now but if you don't, this seems a fitting time to tell you, that life is changing for us all. Luke and Zinnie and I are planning a new adventure, and moving to Canada."

I scan the room when Julie says this and see the odd surprised face, but I guess that it's not news anymore.

"It means that Alice and I are having to sell up and I can't tell you how painful that is for me – firstly to be saying goodbye to Amethi, but most of all that Luke's and my decision is the driver for this. I promise you, Alice," Julie says, taking my hand and looking into my eyes, "I could have happily lived and worked the rest of my life at Amethi with you." She gulps, and I sob.

"Get a room, you two!" Luke says loudly, lightening the mood.

"Although tonight is meant to be about me and Luke," Julie says, "I think it also is about Alice, and her friendship, and love, and generosity. She is a cornerstone in my life. She has been since we were eleven years old, and she always will be, wherever I am. I just want to say such a huge thank you to you, Alice. For tonight, and for everything. To Alice."

I had not foreseen a moment when everybody gathered would be raising their glasses to me, and it makes me catch my breath. I lean shyly into Julie, feeling like Zinnia leaning into Luke. There is a round of applause, and then I scurry across the room to Lydia, who is smiling at me, and is thankfully organised, bringing structure back to the evening. Because there is a further surprise in store. Luke swears loudly when he sees the band come into the room. They've been waiting patiently outside while we made our speeches, and now they are moving in while Lydia's staff politely and efficiently move the furniture around so that there is now space for not only the band but a dance floor too.

"That's not... Skaburst?" Luke asks, practically jumping for joy.

"It is," I confirm.

"No way!"

I put my arm round him. "For you, Luke."

"Alice, I love you!" He hugs me tightly and swings me around then he drags me onto the floor as the band starts up. I reach out a hand for Julie. "You two are meant to have the first dance!"

I have requested that the first song is a fittingly romantic one. I have asked for Madness *It Must Be Love*, though I don't know if it's something that would normally be on a set list. As the band start up, I join Luke's and Julie's hands together, and Luke pulls his wife towards him, kissing her and grinning. Guests gather and applaud them, before joining them on the dance floor as well, and soon, as the tempo increases to more upbeat, bouncier numbers, the room is filled with noise, from the band and from feet on the dance floor.

"I'm scared the floor's going to give way!" Lydia grins when I make my way out of the throng to find a drink.

"Let's hope not." I raise my glass to her. "Thank you so much for letting us do this here. It's just turning out to be the best evening ever."

"It's my pleasure. And I'm really glad to see you and Julie back to normal."

"Me too."

"And Alice, I did want to talk to you, about our conversation, about Amethi—"

"Don't worry," I interrupt her, not wanting to get into work talk now. "I completely understand." Over Lydia's shoulder, I see a group of people looking in through the double doors.

"Oh no," I say. It's the group from Amethi, the one with that Rupert bloke. I hope he's not going to try anything on with Lydia tonight.

Lydia follows my line of vision. "Oh no," she echoes.

"I'll tell them to go to the bar," I say.

"No, I'd better. And I'd better get Si, too."

"Si?" I ask, surprised.

"Yes. That's Xavier."

"What?"

"Xavier. His agent."

Xavier. That's the guy who I had heard being called Zed earlier. Surely Ex would make more sense. Maybe his friends can't spell. But that's not important right now.

"What are they doing here?" I ask, annoyed.

"I think I know," Lydia says grimly. "Don't worry, Alice. You go and enjoy the party, we've got this covered. I won't let them in here."

She goes across to them and I look for Si, but I can see he's already on his way. I want to know what's going on, and I want to know if I can help, but this is Luke and Julie's night, and soon they won't be around anymore. I watch long enough to see Si speaking angrily to his agent, and then the whole group head back out of the room, to who knows where.

As I lose myself in the pure joy of dancing to great music, surrounded by great people, I almost forget all about those unwelcome guests. I catch sight of Si and Lydia dancing, too, so I guess they've given Xavier and Rupert their marching orders. Even so, Lydia doesn't let her hair down for long, keeping her professional, responsible head firmly screwed on.

When I finally take a breather, I see David heading towards me.

"You're a class act, Alice Branvall."

"Why thank you!" The drink and the dancing has gone to my head.

"To you," he says.

"To me," I agree, grinning. "And to you, and Bea, and

the Sail Loft. How's it going?"

"Oh, it's… we've had a few little arguments, but you know what we're like. Seriously, it's so exciting! This time last year, I'd never have imagined I'd be doing this."

"I know. Life's kind of brilliant sometimes, isn't it?"

"Do you know what? Yes it, is. Never mind this time last year, in fact. Just think back to this time ten years ago! You thought you and Sam were over. Now look at you."

We both watch Sam, who is dancing and laughing with Luke. I feel awash with love for him, and I remember how he was in the morning; how he's been feeling about things. I've been so embroiled in my own feelings, and with trying to get things sorted for the party, and for the sale of Amethi, I have not been thinking nearly enough about him. I make a mental promise to myself to do much better.

"It's a lesson, isn't it?" I say. "An important one, at that. Things change. You can feel like you've reached the very bottom of things but if you keep trudging along, you can get to a point where you've risen again, and you can look back at what you've just come through. I think if you can remember that you will get to that point, you'll be OK. But sometimes people just don't have it in themselves to realise that they will get there."

"And sometimes people almost don't want to," David says. "I've been so worried about Bea since Bob died. She's had some terrible moments, which I know she wouldn't want me to share with you, but I've been properly worried about her."

"It will be so good for her, working with you. It will be amazing for both of you!" I say. "I'm so happy for you, David."

"I'm just sorry I couldn't take up your offer of coming to Amethi as well," he says. "I'm gutted for you that you have to leave."

"I think I've come to accept it now," I say, and I look across to Julie, who is holding hands with Holly and dancing. "God, I'm going to miss her."

"I know." David puts his arm around me. "I know."

But as I sit for a moment and just survey the scene, I consider how transient life is, and that things do change – sometimes for the better and sometimes for the worse, but they always change. And maybe Julie and I would have grown tired of Amethi. I would not have chosen to end things yet, but at least we haven't had the chance to let things grow tired and stale – or to let difficult finances begin to change things so that it became a constant worry rather than a joy. This way, I think, we are going out on a high.

24

A couple of weeks after the party, Sam and I head to Paul and Shona's, for the lunch Paul had suggested. When we pull up, there is an expensive-looking car on the drive. I have no idea what it is, but Sam clearly does. He gives a low whistle. "Paul's clearly not suffering in the cost-of-living crisis," he says.

"Well no, but we knew that anyway," I say, feeling slightly spiky around the subject of Paul, as I often do. Sam has never said he has a problem with the fact that Paul and I had a relationship of sorts, and I don't really think that he has. In truth, it never really got off the ground anyway, but the two of them are very different in many ways, and particularly materially. Would Sam want Paul's wealth? Not necessarily, although it would certainly make life a lot easier for us in many ways. I just sometimes think there is an edge of disapproval there, but I could be imagining it.

We park next to the shiny black car, and I can't help but wish we'd washed ours. There is seagull poo on the bonnet which, as Dad regularly tells us, will damage the paintwork if we don't clean it off.

Ben and Holly were invited, but I wasn't sure how strong that invitation was: "Bring the littlies if you think they'd like to come," Shona had said.

Paul's children have grown up and long since flown the nest, both living in London now, and doing very well for themselves ("It helps that Daddy's got a bit of cash and lots of connections," Sam has said a little snidely). I suppose the thought of two small, loud, messy children may not fit in with Shona's idea of a relaxing, social Sunday lunch.

Mum and Dad are looking after Holly and Ben at our house, which they will enjoy much more anyway. Dad seems to have recovered some of his energy these days – probably just from not being worn out by work – and he's certainly happy to share it with the kids, playing silly games with them. I watched him last week, getting them to jump across the cushions he had laid out in the lounge and hallway of the bungalow, while he pretended to be a crocodile intent on catching them for his tea. They were both squealing with an equal mix of terror and joy. It was so good to see him back to something like his normal self. So Ben and Holly are happy, and for my part, coming out for a grown-up meal cooked by somebody else feels really good.

"Alice! Sam!" Shona is at the front door, smiling and looking incredibly glamorous, not a hair out of place as usual. She is much better suited to Paul than I am.

She hugs us both and apologises for being 'such a mess'.

"Oh yeah," I say, "you look terrible."

She laughs. "I do love you, Alice."

"Thanks."

"Now, I forgot to mention we've invited another couple…"

Oh no. Thoughts of a nice, chilled lunch immediately evaporate. I do like to be sociable but sometimes it's nice to just be with people that you already know.

"Hi Alice!" Lydia appears in the hallway, and Si joins her. Phew. This is a surprise, but a relief. I am quite happy to hang out with these two.

"Lydia!" I say, hugging her, then greeting Si with a kiss on the cheek. Shona asks Sam and me what we'd like to drink and then we follow Lydia through to the lounge area. I remember it so well, this house. I was in awe of it when I came here so many years ago, and I still am. It's like something you'd see on TV, with no expense spared, and incredible attention to detail. Not to mention the huge windows framing a view of the sea, and the woods which lead down to the little beach below.

"Hi Sam." Paul stands and shakes Sam's hand, then he hugs me and kisses me on the cheek. His skin is smooth and cool, and he smells of some kind of expensive aftershave. "Hello you," he says. I forgot to mention he can be a tiny bit cheesy. And I think he likes the fact that there was once something between us. But I know he and Shona are very happy together, and he wouldn't mess her about. I don't think he'd dare. I know I wouldn't.

"I hope you don't mind us crashing your lunch," Lydia says, as Shona comes through with the drinks. I have a gin & tonic, and Sam has a zero-alcohol beer. There are bowls of pistachio nuts and olives on the table. I sit down, putting my icy-cold glass on a coaster, and help myself to some nuts.

Sam wanders over to have a look through the window.

"Of course we don't mind!" I say. "It's great to see you. Thanks again for making the party such a great night."

"It was my pleasure. Did Julie and Luke enjoy themselves?"

"So much!"

"That's fab. I'm so pleased."

I had almost forgotten about Si getting annoyed at Xavier that night. I wonder what happened there. He looks a lot happier now, as he sits down next to Lydia and puts his arm around her. She looks happy, too. It's good to see.

"That your new motor on the drive, Paul?" Sam asks.

"My...? Oh, no, you mean the R8? No, that's Si's."

"Ahh," says Sam. "That makes sense. Nice wheels, Si," he says.

"Thanks! Do you want to come and have a look?"

"Si!" Lydia exclaims. "Who are you, Jeremy Clarkson?"

"No, I'd love to," Sam says. I'm surprised, I didn't think he was really into cars, but maybe it taps into a boyhood interest.

"Paul?" Si asks.

"My god, this really is the 1970s!" laughs Shona. "The women stay in gossiping while the men go and look at the posh car."

"You're welcome to come and have a look too...?" Si suggests.

"No thanks," says Shona, and we all laugh. The three men disappear off together, and I sink back into my seat.

"Well," Shona says, "this actually might be a good opportunity, with them out of the way, to have a little chat."

"Oh yes?" I wonder what's coming.

"Yes. Well, I was going to talk to you about this at some point, Alice. It's part of the reason for inviting you, although of course we've been meaning to do this for ages anyway. I've got some news, you see."

"Go on."

Lydia is sitting back, shelling pistachio nuts. It seems she already knows whatever this news is.

"Well, I'm having a bit of an overhaul, career-wise."

"Really?"

"Yes. I'm – I'm giving something new a go."

"Oh, wow. I thought you loved PR."

"I do. I do, and I don't want to give it up completely, but I, well…" She looks at Lydia, who nods. "I'm going to be Si's agent."

"No!"

"Yes! It's absolute madness. I haven't done anything quite like it before and I still cannot believe he's entrusting me with it, but—"

"But Xavier is a wanker!" Lydia laughs.

"Very much so," agrees Shona.

"But this is strictly, strictly between us at the moment," Lydia says. "In fact, I know this is a really difficult thing to do, but could you perhaps not even tell Sam please, just for the time being? There's loads of legal stuff to sort out. Including Si getting out of the film in the US."

"Does he not want to do it?"

"No, or he says he doesn't. I've made him promise he's not giving up on it for me. But he says it's too tied up with Xavier, and that he wants to be close to home anyway. His sister's just had twins, and his mum and dad are kind of old parents anyway. He's quite a family man," she says proudly. "And he's got loads of work opportunities over here. Shona's just getting to grips with them all, aren't you, Shona?"

"Aye, and it's not easy, I can tell you, Alice. I like the challenge, though. I haven't pushed myself like this for a long, long time."

"I can imagine."

"But like I say, I don't want to let the PR stuff go entirely. I mean, I don't like to say this in front of Lydia, but this might not work out."

Lydia laughs. "Si and Shona have agreed on a two-year contract, to see how it goes," she says to me.

"That seems sensible."

"Shona wasn't sure at first, were you? But seriously, Shona, knowing what Xavier was like – a supreme bullshitter – I know you're going to be great."

"Thanks very much!" Shona laughs.

Lydia's cheeks flush. "No, no, I mean, you're the opposite. You may not have the same contacts Xavier does, but you're brilliant at making contacts, at negotiating, at details…"

"I knew what you meant," Shona says, smiling. "Thank you, Lydia. To you and Si, for having faith in me. I'm so excited about all this!"

"So what about your existing business?" I ask.

"Well, that's where you come in. If you'd like to…"

Shona goes on to outline how she would like somebody to take over the day-to-day running of the business. "Maybe do some writing, too – press releases, that kind of thing. If you'd like to, Alice. I've always liked the way you work, and I know you're looking for something different. I also know you've got a lot going on with the family at the moment. I will not be at all offended if you say no, but I would love it if you did."

"Wow," I say, genuinely taken aback. "I was not expecting that. Any of it," I laugh. "That's amazing about you taking on Si's stuff."

"Remember nobody else can know about it yet," Lydia says, as though we could be being listened to, even now.

"Don't worry," I reassure her. "And Shona, thank you so much. That really does sound like an amazing opportunity. I... can I think about it?"

"Well, yes, of course! And there is no rush. Why don't we get together, just the two of us, for lunch, maybe the week after next? That should give you time to think of lots of questions, and we'll hopefully have more news about the – other thing – by then as well."

"Brilliant. Thank you." My head is swimming with thoughts and I'm already imagining what it might be like to do something so different. And what it could be like to work for Shona. She and I get on very well, and I like the way she works. Also, while she is a friend, we are not close enough that I would worry about anything workwise affecting our friendship. I've been there and done that with my best friend and I think the way forward now is to keep things strictly business.

"So how's the Amethi sale going?" Shona asks.

"Ah well, that's predictably complicated," I say. "But I know Peter's a friend of Paul's."

"Maybe of Paul's, but not of mine," Shona says quickly.

"Oh?"

"Not a fan," she says. "Not that that should have any bearing on your selling to him. I just find him a bit..."

"Sneaky?" I say, before I've even thought about which

word is going to come out of my mouth. The truth is, he's been chipping away at his offer, ever since we first agreed that he would buy up. I kind of knew this would happen, but not to the extent that it has. We agreed a price based on various conditions and Julie and I have been very open and amenable when it's come to him sending various people round to check over the properties, utilities, drains, etc, but all of these people seem to find a lot of faults with them. And each of these faults leads to a reduction in the offer price. It's starting to drive me and Julie mad, and our visions of leaving the business with anything to our names at all are evaporating fast.

I explain all this and Shona and Lydia listen sympathetically. I can see Lydia is a little on edge and I feel bad in case it's because she turned down my offer to become my partner.

"Can I freshen up your drinks, girls?" Shona asks. It's been a while since anyone called me a girl, and a fleeting memory springs to mind, of a man calling me and Julie girls when we headed down to the beach that first night we'd come back down to Cornwall. Even then, I'd felt too old, but it's a long time ago now, and it certainly feels it.

"Alice..." Lydia says, almost timidly, when Shona has bustled off to the kitchen.

"Yes?"

"I wanted to talk to you about something. About... Amethi."

"Please don't say you've changed your mind about coming to work with me!" I laugh. Her face turns red again. Oh no. I really don't know what I'll say if that's what she wants to do.

I've made peace with the idea of moving on now. And I've realised there is a kind of relief at the thought of being less torn when it comes to family things. Besides, Shona has just made me that job offer, and it's got me thinking.

"No, not exactly." She clears her throat, and sits straighter, and I see the professional Lydia come to the fore. "No, it's… I don't know if it's too late, if you're too far down the road with this other guy, but Si and I would like to make you an offer. For Amethi. For the whole thing."

"You'd…?"

"We've been talking, a lot. And we want to make changes. I hate, hate, hate having people snooping on us, and having to watch what I say all the time. And I feel like I've done as much as I can at the Bay."

"You've done brilliantly," I say.

"Thank you," she smiles shyly, but resumes her professional, serious manner. "We'd like to take it on, Amethi, and carry on running it the way that you and Julie do. I mean, I need a chef, but I think I can poach Tristan from the Bay, and if I can't, I know lots of other people. And Si will be away a lot, filming, but hopefully mostly in the UK instead of the States. So he won't be much use! I think I've worked it out, though, how we'd do it, and I wanted to run it all past you to see what you think. If you're open to the idea," she says, a note of doubt slipping in again.

"Well," I say slowly, "I'd have to talk to Julie, of course."

"Of course."

"And we are, as you know, somewhere down this slippery path with this Peter guy, but he's the one making problems for us, so I don't know that he's really got a leg to stand on.

Shit," I say. "I love the idea of you taking it on. I need to talk to Julie!"

Suddenly, I'm a bundle of energy and nerves, and I want to get moving, but we have come for lunch, and it's Sunday, and Julie and Luke and Zinnia are up at Cherry's today anyway, trying to make sure they spend as much time with her as they can before they leave the country.

Shona returns with our glasses, and she's smiling. "Have you two had a chance to talk?"

"Yes, we… you knew?"

"Yes of course, this is exactly the kind of thing my new client should be talking to me about," she grins. "But I am not going to ask what you think. I know there's a lot to talk about with Julie. And I know you'll want to talk to Sam as well, about my job offer. Just don't mention what I'm planning to do instead, though. Just for the time being."

"Yes, yes, I get the message!" I laugh. "You can trust me."

"We know we can," they say together, and I laugh again.

We have a delicious lunch, and there is plenty of wine flowing along with the conversation. Si keeps us entertained with stories from the world of showbiz, although I notice he is careful not to give anyone's identity away. I don't normally drink at lunchtime, and I can feel my face is flushed, from the alcohol and from all the new, unexpected ideas which are flooding my mind.

"You were on good form," Sam says as he drives us back.

"Was I?"

"Yeah! It was like having the old Alice back," he says. "Though I didn't really realise she'd gone anywhere. But I know it's been tough for you lately."

"It has," I agree, but I really don't want to get any further into that side of things. I want to maintain this positivity. "Shona offered me a job," I say.

"She what?" He glances over at me. Only briefly, because we are on one of those slender lanes with tall hedges banking either side of it. I am glad he's driving.

"Yeah. She's branching out a bit, and she wants me to come and work for her."

"And… do you want to?" He is being cautious, but I know it would be a great relief to Sam – and to me – to know that I already have another source of income sorted.

"Do you know what? I think I do! There is lots to think about, but I like the idea."

"Well, that's amazing!"

As we come onto a wider road, Sam pulls off into a layby. It's actually a place I'd stopped with Paul once, in the summer, and we'd got chips from a van that was parked here. I don't mention that now.

"Why are we stopping here?" I ask instead.

Sam pulls the car into a space so that it is facing out to sea. It's only late afternoon but it's nearly dark, and the lighthouse is already flashing its warning to anyone looking. Dark, moody clouds are moving quickly, and the water looks distinctly unsettled.

"I just wanted to make the most of this bit of time, just me and you," Sam says.

I look at him, and feel a rush of love. "I am so lucky," I smile.

"*We* are so lucky," he says. "Me, you, and the kids. We have each other."

"We do." I think of Julie, and how pissed off I've been at her, unfairly, because of her wanting to do the right thing for her family. What would I do, if Sam wanted to move abroad? Or not even abroad – just somewhere else? Not that it's all Luke's idea, to go to Canada, but I know his grief has been a driving factor in them assessing their lives. If you want to be in a relationship, and if you have a family, then it has to be about compromise sometimes, and working things out for the best for all of you. Besides, as Lizzie wisely tried to point out, Cornwall was always my dream, not Julie's. Maybe I should have always known that there would come a time when she'd want to move on. "We do," I say again, "and I wouldn't change a thing."

"Not even diabetes?" He looks at me earnestly.

"Well, yes. I would. I would change that. If one of us had to have it, I would take it myself. But we can't change it and we have to make the best of it, and make sure Holly does, too. I know it won't be easy." I've already more than once leapt ahead to Holly's teenage years, and can foresee potential issues there, but that is a long way ahead. I have to learn to take things as they come.

"I wouldn't let you. I'd have it," Sam says. "I'd have the diabetes."

And we actually collapse into laughter as the conversation has begun to sound ridiculous. I wipe a tear from my eye and for once it's from happiness. Then I unclip my seatbelt, and I lean across and kiss my husband on the lips. Firmly, and satisfyingly.

"Steady on," he murmurs, but he kisses me back, and we lose ourselves for a while. Just me and Sam in the peace and solitude of the car, in the dark. Sam unclips his seatbelt so he can put his arms around me, and he strokes my hair then twists his fingers into it as he kisses me. "I love you, Alice. So much."

"I love you too," I say. "So, so much."

"Alright, it's not a competition," he smiles as he leans his forehead against mine. "Better not get too carried away up here anyway… we'll get into trouble."

"Shame," I smile, but in truth the kiss was perfect. A reconnection between us. We sit for just a few moments longer, feeling happy and content, and watching the last remnants of light drip from the sky.

Humming, Sam drives us home, and my heart leaps at the sight of our house – our home – lights on in the midst of the winter darkness. We pull onto the drive and kiss once more, just briefly, before we get out of the car and head inside. It is warm when we open the door and Meg trots happily up to greet us. Meanwhile, there are voices and laughter coming from the kitchen and I go in to find Mum has cooked tea for everyone.

"I hope you don't mind," she says. "Ben said he was starving."

"And me, Mummy," Holly says.

"Yes, and they both helped me work out the carbs for Holly," Dad says proudly.

"Well that's brilliant!" I smile and kiss each of them in turn.

"Did you have a nice time?" Mum asks.

"Yes, it was great thanks."

"Well, you deserve a break. Shall I put the kettle on? Make us all a cup of tea?"

"That would be lovely. Thanks, Sue," says Sam.

"Go on, you two, you go and sit down. We've got everything covered here."

"Ah, thank you, Mum. You are brilliant."

"I know."

We do as we are told, and we go into the lounge. I tuck my legs up onto the seat, and lean against Sam while he puts his arm around me. Once the kids have finished their tea, they bound in and demand we play with them. "Jumping Monkeys!" shouts Holly. It's her favourite game right now.

Go on then!" I smile. She pulls the box out, and Ben gets a pile more.

"Are we playing all of these?" I ask.

"Yep!"

Dad brings through a tray of tea and biscuits and we settle in for the evening, all of us relaxed and happy. We have such a laugh. It feels like a really long time since we've been like this. Sometimes you really don't realise you've missed something until you find it again.

25

It is New Year's Eve. The last day of a very, very eventful year. Also the day of David and Martin's party. It seems to have swung round very fast.

I have had Bea on the phone to me nearly every day – always apologetic, but always on the phone, or so it seems. Still, in this situation, she is a client, and I treat her exactly as I would any other customer. She just needs lots of reassurance – that everything is in hand, and that she is doing the right thing.

"Julie and Luke didn't mind being surprised, did they?" she has asked me about thirty times.

"No, Bea, they loved it! And honestly, I have no doubts that David will. Or Martin."

It's Martin she's worried about, I can tell. David, she knows inside-out. She is a bit older than him, so after their parents both died, she kind of took on a mothering role, but he is equally protective of her.

"Look, Martin's parents love the idea, don't they? If anyone knows what Martin would like – besides David, I mean – it will be them," I say, hoping that it's true and knowing that actually parents aren't always the best people to know what their children want. Even so, this is a lovely thing that Bea is doing, and I really am sure that both David and Martin will be touched beyond words.

"What about it being New Year's Eve? Will people mind, do you think?"

"Bea!" I laugh. "It's a bit late for that now!"

I (politely) end the call and then Julie and I go around the Mowhay, checking that all the twinkly little battery-powered lights Lizzie left us are working, and double-checking the table settings. Bea has asked for a sit-down meal, and she's devised the seating plan. She will be sitting with David, Martin, Tyler, Esme, and David's parents. She has put me and Julie and our families on the next table. I'm taking this as a compliment, rather than it being for easy access in case she needs us to do anything.

"Here, watch this," Julie says, pretending to blow out one of the little candles, timing the switch-off perfectly.

"Idiot!" I laugh.

"You're just jealous of my magic powers."

"True. You've got nothing on Lizzie, though," I say. "I do miss her."

"I know. Me too. It sounds like she's having the time of her life, though."

Lizzie has kept in touch more frequently than I'd thought she would – she emails Julie and me together, and sends us lots of pictures of the places she and Med are staying, or sites they have visited. Sometimes she sends pictures of the two of them. She looks happy.

"I've… had… the time of my life——" I begin to sing but Julie rudely interrupts me.

"No! We are not having *Dirty Dancing* songs. Only classy music, Bea said so."

247

"But Bea's not here."

"Nevertheless, we start as we mean to go on."

I can feel a bubbling up of childish liveliness in me and I can tell Julie is just the same. We have always fed off each other's energy like this, and when there's an event at our children's school, we seem to revert to our schoolgirl selves, and become very silly and giggly.

"We'll have to split you up," Luke had said at the Christmas service, all teacherly-sternness. "You clearly can't be trusted."

That had only made us worse.

We have already promised ourselves and each other to focus on the positives, and try not to think about what the day marks for Amethi and our lives here. Because after the party, and after the current holiday-makers have headed home, taking their New Year's hangovers with them, Amethi will step into its annual January slumber, closing for the month, and when it comes out the other side, it will be Lydia who is running it.

I am so pleased that it's her, and that we managed to pull out of negotiations with Peter, who was not best pleased, but shouldn't have messed us about so much. Lydia already has her army of staff sorted, and an incredible business plan, of which I feel a little bit jealous. She will honour all the current holiday bookings, but she is going to build on this place being a retreat, and an event location. Yoga, writing, art and music weeks. Quiet weeks for creative people to hole themselves away in a beautiful place, knowing that they will be fed and watered at regular intervals. She has some ready-made contacts via Si, although I know she is determined not to rely too much on them. I can just see it now, and I know it will work so well. While I wish I could be a part of it, I am also looking forward to my new job, with Shona, which I start in March. I have two months, ostensibly to help Lydia with the handover, but I am also hoping to find a little bit of space to myself somewhere in there.

By the time I begin my own new role, Julie, Luke and Zinnia will be in Toronto. They leave at the end of January, and already their home here is taking on that 'up in the air' feeling. I certainly cannot think about that now. The one thing keeping me, and I think all of us, from panicking about it is that they are not selling up. They are renting their house to a family from school, and I think knowing that they will still have a firm place here is a comfort to us all.

Anyway, today is not a day to get maudlin about these things. It is a day of celebration.

By six o'clock, Julie and I have changed into our evening dresses. Bea had wanted the event to be black-tie, and I am sure that her brother and his husband will approve. She's got tuxedos for David and Martin, which she has taken with her when she's gone to collect them. She's telling them that we are all partying together, and starting with a drink at the Mowhay, to say goodbye to Amethi.

"It's quite handy you're selling up," she said, "it gives me the perfect excuse to get them up here."

"Thanks, Bea," I had replied with some meaning in my voice.

"Oh, erm, yes, sorry, Alice. That was a bit insensitive of me."

"You think?" I'd said, but I'd smiled. "It will work perfectly."

I am starting to feel the nerves myself, knowing that Bea is on her way. She's told Tyler and Esme, who are old enough to keep a secret, although apparently Esme's been so excited, she's nearly given it away more than once. Bea has also invited Tyler's girlfriend, Annie, which is lovely of her. Annie has arrived already, looking young and beautiful in a black dress, and is sitting nervously by the door. Julie goes over to her, and I see her make Annie laugh. It makes my stomach twist, I feel so much love for my friend. I can't let myself go there now, though.

"Sshhh… sshhh… they're here!" Dad hisses, from his vantage point by the bifold doors. A whisper goes round the room, and everyone hushes.

I smile to myself, hearing David's animated voice from outside.

"Hope he's not slagging any of us off," Julie whispers in my ear.

"Sshhh!" I say, suppressing the urge to giggle.

"Ho-ly shit!" David says, as he walks in, cut off mid-sentence, and clearly genuinely flabbergasted by the sight before him.

"What?" Martin, a step behind, asked, having to stop himself from walking into the back of his husband. "Jesus, Mary and Joseph!"

"Don't forget the donkey!" somebody calls, and the room erupts with laughter as people's pent-up emotions are let loose.

"Surprise!" I shout, somewhat redundantly.

"No shit, Sherlock!" says David. He comes towards me, looking incredibly handsome in his black-tie gear – Martin possibly even more so.

"You make quite the couple," I say.

"Damn right we do," David says, kissing Martin on the cheek.

Martin responds by kissing David on the lips. Then he hugs Bea. "This is all your doing, is it?"

"Well, yes, but with quite a truckload of help from Alice and Julie!"

"Thank you, ladies." Julie and I accept kisses off both the happy couple.

Bea takes her brother and Martin by the hand and leads them around, showing them the seating plan, and making them stop to speak to each guest in turn. Sam is on music duty and now that the guests of honour have arrived, he starts his specially selected playlist, beginning with Louis Armstrong singing *La Vie en Rose*.

"We'll never get to eat at this rate," I say, but Julie is a step ahead of me. She bangs a spoon on the big wooden table.

"Ladies and gentlemen, please take your seats!" she says. "Dinner is about to be served."

"About time too!" shouts Ron, and Karen, already a sheet or two to the wind, tries to shush him.

"That's enough from you, Ronald," calls Julie. "If you want to eat, you'll sit down…"

"And keep my mouth shut?" he calls jovially.

"Exactly."

As people begin to take their seats, I do a quick check of the tables to make sure that there are bottles of wine and jugs of water on each. The chatter subsides as the waiting staff – including Sophie and her friend Amber, who chose to work and get paid double-time rather than attend the party, which apparently is for old crumblies anyway – serve each table in turn.

There are generous bowls of pasta with creamy tomato and mascarpone sauce, or seafood risotto. Side bowls of crisp salad and mini tins of individual servings of focaccia. Large bottles of olive oil, chilli oil, rosemary oil, and balsamic vinegar sit alongside the wine. "Let's hope nobody gets those mixed up," says Sam.

As everybody tucks into their food, I glance around the room. I see that Julie is doing the same. It's customary anyway, to make sure everything is as it should be, but tonight I have another thought in my mind, that this is the last event we will be hosting here. I am quite sure Julie's thinking along the same lines.

I catch David's eye, and he smiles at me, mouthing 'Thank you', and raising his glass. I lift mine in return.

It is a genuine thrill to see him and Martin together, with their family, from Martin's lovely, slightly shy dad, to Esme. Bea appears to be holding court, which is as I would expect, but I am struck not for the first time by just how brave and strong that woman is. I'm so glad she's back in the Sail Loft. It was lovely having Mum and Dad there, but it feels like things have slotted back into place now, and are just as they should be.

After the palate-cleansing sorbet, and before the dessert of lemon or chocolate torte – both made with the crumbliest, sweetest, short pastry, and doused with as much cream as desired – Bea stands to address the whole room.

"Thank you so very much for coming, and spending your valuable New Year's Eve with us," she smiles around genially. "I can't tell you how much it means to me, that you've made the effort, and I am sure that Martin and my little brother David feel the same. Now, as many of you will know, their actual anniversary was a couple of weeks back, but rather selfishly, they had already made plans for that night. In fact, Martin was whisking David away for a romantic getaway, and thankfully he had entrusted me with that secret some time ago – so I knew I would have to find another date for their party. Really, what better night than New Year's Eve? It's about endings; it's about beginnings. It's about celebrating what has been, and anticipating what is to come. For David and me, that will be welcoming guests to *our* hotel. And I cannot wait to be working with my brother. He knows me better than anyone and I like to think that, after Martin, I hold the same position for David." I see him nodding, and reaching for her hand. "But while we are on the subject of Martin, I would just like to say how incredibly happy I am that he and David are together. I honestly don't think I know a more perfect couple, and I know some pretty perfect ones!" She smiles over at our table. Julie and I grin at each other, while Luke and Sam both look pleased but a bit embarrassed. "I know how hard it is to find real, lasting love, and not just that but a true partnership. When I look at David and Martin, I see all of that. And more. They're inspirational parents, and I know Tyler and Esme realise just how lucky they are to have them—"

"Even if they don't always show it," David says, just loud

enough for everyone to hear, and he ruffles Esme's hair. She looks at once delighted and mortified, if that is possible.

"You remember what I was like as a teenager?" Bea asks David and he looks mock-horrified. "Exactly! Think yourself lucky! Anyway, what I am getting at here is just how lucky I am – we are – to have these two gentlemen in our lives. Without David and Martin, and their wonderful children, I honestly don't know if I would have made it through this last year or two."

She finally cracks, and she's not the only one. I squeeze Sam's hand, and see there is a quiet teardrop rolling down his cheek.

I suspect it makes us all think, of how lucky we are. I know that Dad is thinking of Mum, and how she almost died a few years back; she, I am sure, will be thinking of how ill he has been thanks to covid, and how so many other people were even more unlucky. Julie, perhaps, will be thinking of Luke's recent state of mind, and how he's pulled himself back from the brink. I remember Sam's cliffside accident, and how he had to be rescued from the rocks. It could have ended so differently. I can't even bear to think of what would have happened to Holly if we hadn't realised when we did that she was diabetic. I want to hug Sam and our children to me, and at the same time I want to go up and hug Bea. David and Martin take that honour, though, all three of them with tears running down their faces. After a few quiet moments, there is a gradual smattering of applause, which grows into something bigger, and louder, and stronger. Martin and David stand back and Martin insists that Bea, now laughing through her tears, takes a bow.

"Thank you, everyone," David says, when the room has grown quiet. "I can only echo what Bea has said, about how very special it is that you have chosen to share this evening with us. And I also would like to thank Martin, my wonderful, supportive, and drop-dead-gorgeous husband." There is a whoop from the back of the room. I look and I think I see Lydia grinning at Si. Was it him? If it was, I like him even more.

But it also hits me again, that soon this place will be theirs. I am glad – so glad – knowing that it will be in good hands, but even so… Still, tonight is not about me. Not by a long way.

"Ten years sounds like such a long time," David continues, and I admire his capacity for speaking like this, completely unplanned. "And yet no time at all. In this last ten years, we have gained Tyler and Esme. And in another ten years, they'll be in their early twenties, doing who knows what? It goes by in a flash, really it does, so if I could say anything to you all – and I know I am not exactly renowned for my worldly advice – it is to cherish as many moments as you can. Stop, and think about things as and when they happen. I don't mean everything. I don't even mean every day. But try and recognise the important times, whether it's getting married, or it's cuddling your kids while you watch a film together. One day, they'll be too big for that kind of thing, or they'll be miles away, across the world. It's all good, it's all great. Nothing can stay the same, and people will grow as they should – if they're lucky," he says, looking at Bea. "I think living here, by the sea, we're extra aware of the way things constantly change. The weather, the tide, the sand… it may look the same, but it is always shifting. Sometimes imperceptibly, sometimes it's blown into huge, great drifts. Marriage is a bit like that, too. And love. But, at the risk of sounding incredibly cheesy, how I feel about Martin never changes – or, if it does, it only gets better, and stronger. Ten years is a drop in the ocean, but I am so glad I've spent them with him. Martin, my love, I hope that we have many more."

Martin stands and hugs David and they rock each other back and forth a little. I steal a glance at Tyler, who has his arm around Annie, and looks proud. Esme is clearly trying not to cry, and Bea puts her arm around her.

What a night. I don't know if I can take any more emotion! Thankfully, Julie reads things well, and she heads off to summon the waiting staff, to bring out the dessert, followed by pots of tea and coffee, and little trays of chocolates.

Sam takes his cue and goes to put the music back on, this time a little louder and more upbeat, the first track the Black-Eyed Peas' *I Gotta Feeling*, and then Paul and Shona are up on the dance floor, with no prompting. It gets a few other people up, too, and soon there are more people dancing than sitting.

"Shall we?" says Sam.

"You never dance!"

"I do tonight. Make the most of it." He takes Holly by the hand as well, and I grab Ben, and we dance, the four of us, then form a wider circle as Julie and Zinnia, then Luke, join us. And as the children grow tired, Mum and Dad whisk them away, so that the four of us can enjoy the rest of the night.

Sophie comes to join in, too, once the washing-up is done. But she has an ulterior motive. "Can Amber and me go into town now?" she asks.

"Yes," Sam says. "Of course. I don't think David and Martin would mind."

"Hey, we're just the hired help!" Sophie grins. "They're not allowed to mind."

"You're not dressed up," I say, thinking of how the town will be rammed with people in fancy dress tonight.

"Yeah, we're waitresses!" Sophie says, gesturing to their black-and-white dresses. "Or chess pieces, or penguins or something. Anyway, who cares? Everyone will be too pissed by now to notice."

"True. Go on then, have a great time," Sam says.

Just as the girls turn on their heel, I say, "Hang on a minute!"

"What?"

"See you next year!"

"Oh, Alice. So predictable," Sophie says, smiling.

Soon enough, it is midnight. Some of the guests have left before the main moment of the night, having dogs or kids to return to, but there is a good hardcore of us still here. There are the usual suspects, of course: me, Sam, Julie, Luke, David, Martin of course, and Bea. We link arms and sing *Auld Lang Syne* and again I feel keenly how Bea is on her own, but none of us couples feel the need to kiss each other. Instead, we all simultaneously gather in one huge hug, jumping up and down, and wishing each other well, and I find I can't quite look at Julie. Not because I am annoyed at her but because I can't bear to think of what lies ahead. Tonight is a night of celebration, and so I try incredibly hard not to think about what this new year will bring.

257

26

Thanks to the ever-reliable Brian, we manage to get a taxi back to town. David, Martin and Bea are staying at the little cottage at Amethi, and so it is just me, Julie, Sam and Luke who need to get back to town.

We cross paths with some of our guests, who Brian has brought back up here, and we all wish each other well. Dawdling behind as we walk to the car park, I try not to sway as I look up at the stars in the calm, quiet sky. I haven't drunk loads, but it's been more than I would normally at a work function.

A slight breeze rattles the few dry leaves that remain around the feet of the hedgerow. I stop for a moment. *Breathe*, I hear Lizzie's voice and I do as I'm told. A soft, gentle flurry of air fleetingly, tentatively touches my skin, my face and my neck.

"Alice!" I hear.

"Just a moment." I close my eyes and feel it again, over my eyes and my forehead. I imagine it's the spirit, or spirits, of this place. That they are saying goodbye. Even though it won't be the last time I'm here – there is still much to do – but this feels like a momentous occasion. "Thank you," I whisper.

I don't want the others to hear me, or to know what I'm

doing. I open my eyes and I scurry along towards the waiting taxi, clambering into the back, where Sam is wedged in the middle of the seat.

"Alright?" he asks.

"I think so." I lean my head on his shoulder.

As we approach town, and the turning to her road, Julie says, "Wait!"

"What have you forgotten?" I ask.

"No, I mean, do we have to go home right now? The kids are all with your mum and dad, Alice. Shouldn't we make the most of this? I feel like we... we should go to the beach!"

"The beach?" Brian chuckles.

"Yes, the beach," Julie says firmly.

"That's a great idea," I agree, looking across Sam and reaching out for my friend's hand.

"Don't mind me," says Sam, while Brian says, "Customer's always right, they tell me. The beach it is."

"And so, around three hours into this brand-new year, Julie, Luke, Sam and I find ourselves walking barefoot on the sand, where all those years ago we sat together, young and awkward: Luke harbouring unrequited feelings towards Julie; Sam and I sitting either side of them, unsure how to move things on.

Now, we sit again, this time with Julie and me in the middle, Sam to my right and Luke to Julie's left. The tide is a long way out tonight and the moonlight glimmers across the sea and onto the wet sand. Although it is the first day of January, and the middle of the night, it is barely cold.

I push my toes into the sand, feeling the minuscule

grains cascade over my skin. It seems like none of us know what to say.

Sam stands. "I'm going to try a bit of stone-skimming. You coming, Luke?"

Luke stands, brushing the sand off his trousers, and I hear them laughing at something as they head down towards the shore. I envy them their ease, while I just feel churned up again. There have been so many celebrations these last few months, but it feels like such a lot is coming to an end.

"I'm going to miss you so much," I blurt out.

"Oh Alice," Julie leans her head against mine. "We are going to miss you too, you have no idea."

"But we're the ones being left behind," I say, childishly.

"Where you've everyone and everything familiar. All the people you love."

"Not all of them," I say but she doesn't seem to hear. She is looking out to sea, or perhaps towards her husband. I suddenly realise that she is nervous, maybe even scared, about what lies ahead.

"We're going somewhere we've never been, where we don't know anyone."

"So why do it?" I pause. Breathe. "I'm sorry. I know why. And you are doing the right thing, and I think you're going to love it. It must be scary, though."

"It is. It really, truly is, but it feels right. You never know, maybe we'll be back here with our tails between our legs before the year's out."

"You won't. You'll make it work. But if... just if it doesn't, you know where we are."

"I do. Thank you, Alice. And I know it feels like we're

leaving you. Well, we are, but it's not about that. It's what David said, things are ever-changing. I love the way you have always known what you wanted, and I wish I was more like you."

"But I love the way you're open and adventurous. I'm just… just a boring old stick-in-the-mud!" That has us both laughing, and I'm glad. "Come on," I say, "let's go and skim some stones."

I stand, and hold out my hand to Julie. We walk then run down the beach, laughing, and join Sam and Luke at the water's edge. I am absolutely rubbish at skimming stones, and Julie isn't much better. We soon give up. I walk a little way into the sea. The incline here is so gradual, the water is still barely covering my ankles.

"Come and stand with me!" I shout, and obligingly, they do. I take hold of Luke's hand, and then Julie's, and she grabs Sam's.

We stand in a line, looking out across the water and feeling the small waves wash over our feet on their way in and back out again.

"It's cold!" Luke says.

"Don't be a baby," I laugh. "Stand still, and just enjoy it."

I close my eyes and feel their hands in mine, these amazing people who are an essential element of my life and will be no matter where they are. Beneath us, the sea pulls away at the sand so that our feet sink in a little way. I imagine all the tiny creatures burrowed there, sharing their space with us.

Opening my eyes, I see the lights further down the estuary. I scan across the darkness of the water, my eyes searching as far out as they can. I see the lighthouse, and I see… nothing. Or everything. The sea stretches on, and somewhere it meets the sky, but I know that even there it is not the end. I squeeze Luke's hand and Julie's, and without a word, all four of us come together in a hug, laughing as the waves continue to lap around our feet.

"Come on," says Luke. "Time to head back. I'm freezing."

I cast one more glance across the waves, before turning towards the beautiful town where we live; near-empty streets still glittering with Christmas decorations, and ringing with the laughter and shouts of a few stragglers determined to carry on partying, cutting across the echoes of new years past. Who knows what this town has seen in its time? Our story is just one of many.

With the sand gently shifting beneath our feet, we begin to walk forward, together.

Acknowledgements

Well, where do I begin, thinking that this really is, almost certainly, the last book of the Coming Back to Cornwall series, probably. Because as we all know, I've said that before! But I know it has to end somewhere, and I wanted it to have a slightly alternative take on a happy ending. Because as most of us know, there is no such thing as a happy ending – life does not stop at the good parts – and I wanted this book and this series to reflect that. It would be easy as a writer to give characters convenient solutions to problems, but I prefer – sometimes – to find different ways around things, which might require harder work, but will be at least as satisfying.

I owe a lot of thanks to a lot of people for helping me make this series what it is. Firstly, my excellent friend and cover designer, Catherine Clarke. She has not only made my books look beautiful, but she is a very important person to me and all my family. Then there is my dad, Ted Rogers, who is possibly my greatest supporter, and has read and proofread all of these books for me. Which brings me on to Hilary Kerr, who has also been instrumental in proofreading many books in this series and beta reading, and offering excellent editorial advice (as well as sharing her knowledge and experience when it comes to our dogs as well!). I am also incredibly lucky to have a team of super-supportive, generous beta readers, who let me know what they like (or don't like) about a book, and whether or not it works for them as a story. This time round it is thanks to (in no particular order): Rebecca Leech, Sandra Francis, Alison Lassey, Tracey Shaw, Roz Osborne, Mandy Chowney-Andrews, Marilynn Wrigley, Kate Jenkins, Amanda Tudor, Ginnie Ebbrell, Sheila Setter, and Jean Crowe. Author Nelly Harper gets a special mention for putting her own work aside once again to read mine. It is very greatly appreciated.

I also want to say thanks to Skaburst, a real-life band from Telford who kindly allowed me to use their name for Luke and Julie's party entertainment! I thought I'd come up with the name myself, but a quick Google showed me I had no doubt heard it and inadvertently nicked it.

Nicola Collins, friend and PDSN, also deserves a huge THANK YOU for reviewing my diabetes storyline.

When it comes to type one diabetes, my own family has been living alongside it for seven years, since my son was diagnosed at the age of four. When I asked him what he thought about me using it for a storyline, he suggested it might be boring. I hope very much that it hasn't been! I have toyed with the idea of writing about it for a long time as it has such a huge impact on all of our lives. It is a much-misunderstood condition, and those living with it have to consider it in everything they do. But it can, as Alice says, be lived with, and that is what we do – hopefully with as minimal fuss as possible. I am including some information about one of the charities out there, JDRF (Juvenile Diabetes Research Foundation) who work to support those living with diabetes, to make life easier and to one day, hopefully, find a cure. Huge thanks to Edelle Irwin for being so positive and helpful!

To Gill Corbett and Pat Pearce (and Sandra who I have already mentioned) for being my Cornish friends! And to everyone at Redruth Library for your support too.

And thank you, as always, to Chris, Laura and Edward, for being generally brilliant, and for being my family! I am very lucky.

Finally, thanks to my mum and dad, from whom I have inherited my love of books, and for introducing me to Cornwall so many years ago. Who could have imagined then how important it would be to me?

About JDRF and type 1 diabetes

JDRF is the leading global type 1 diabetes charity. We work every day to help people live better with the condition, prevent people ever developing it and one day, find cures. We do this by funding research, campaigning for access to all treatments and connecting and supporting the type 1 community.

Type 1 diabetes is an autoimmune disease that affects both children and adults, regardless of their diet or lifestyle. Over 400,000 people in the UK live with type 1, including 29,000 children. It's unpreventable and at present, there is no cure.

With type 1, your pancreas stops producing insulin, a hormone the body needs to get energy from food. This means a process your body should do naturally and automatically becomes something you must look after yourself, every day. Without this intervention, a person with type 1 would die within a few short days.

With type 1, you must constantly monitor your blood-glucose level. If blood glucose levels are too high or low and left untreated, you will begin to feel unwell. It could lead to serious complications and potentially be fatal. To treat, you must inject or deliver insulin through a pump, carefully balancing these insulin doses with your eating and activity throughout the day and night.

JDRF is driving the acceleration of type 1 research in the UK and across the globe. Significant breakthroughs continue to unlock more knowledge about this condition and cures are closer than ever before. Our work on lab-grown beta cells led to a clinical trial which resulted in someone with type 1 no longer needing to take insulin. JDRF has been the driver behind key research that has brought us to this point.

When we work together, we can achieve incredible things. Together, we can create a world without type 1. A world without finger-prick tests, injections, highs, lows, sleepless nights and disrupted days, where everyone can live their lives to the fullest.

To find out more about JDRF and type 1, please visit
jdrf.org.uk

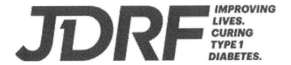

New for winter 2023!

FIRST CHRISTMAS

a novella

and

an introduction to a brand-new series by

Katharine E. Smith.

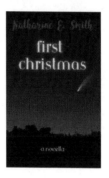

This short, festive story is an exploration of another side of
this time of year normally packed with family, friends and
festivities. It is nevertheless uplifting and engaging, and
full of Christmas spirit.

Coming Back to Cornwall

Books One to Ten

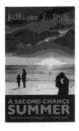

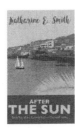

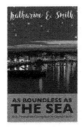

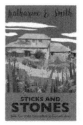

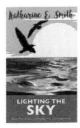

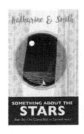

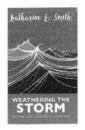

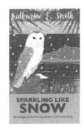

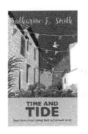

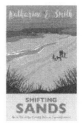

Available in print and on Kindle

The whole Coming Back to Cornwall series is being made into audiobooks so you that you can listen to the adventures of Alice, Julie and Sam while you drive, cook, clean, go to sleep... whatever, wherever!

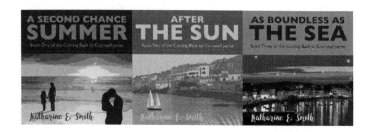

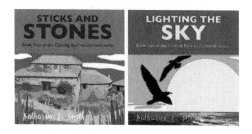

Books One to Five are available now!

Connections

Books One to Three

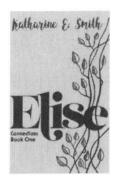

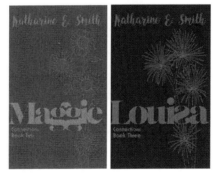

Available in print and on Kindle

Writing the Town Read -
Katharine's first novel. "I seriously couldn't put it down and would recommend it to anyone who doesn't like chick lit, but wants a great story."

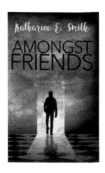

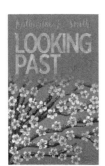

Looking Past - a story of motherhood, and growing up without a mother. "Despite the tough topic the book is full of love, friendships and humour. Katharine Smith cleverly balances emotional storylines with strong characters and witty dialogue, making this a surprisingly happy book to read."

Amongst Friends - a back-to-front tale of friendship and family, set in Bristol.

"An interesting, well written book, set in Bristol which is lovingly described, and with excellent characterisation. Very enjoyable."

Printed in Great Britain
by Amazon

30483519R00160